Medical Management of Chemical Casualties

Fifth Edition

2014

Borden Institute
US Army Medical Department Center and School
Fort Sam Houston, Texas

US Army Medical Research Institute of Chemical Defense
Aberdeen Proving Ground, Maryland

Office of The Surgeon General
United States Army
Falls Church, Virginia

Medical Management of Chemical Casualties Handbook

Borden Institute
Daniel E. Banks, MD, MS, MACP
LTC MC USA
Director and Editor in Chief

Disclaimer: The purpose of this handbook is to provide concise, supplemental reading material for attendees of the Medical Management of Chemical Casualties Course. It is to be used as a guide in the chemical arena and not to replace official doctrine. Every effort has been made to make the information contained in this handbook consistent with official policy and doctrine.

This handbook, however, is not an official Department of the Army publication, nor is it official doctrine. It should not be construed as such unless it is supported by other documents.

Dosage Selection: The authors and publisher have made every effort to ensure the accuracy of dosages cited herein. However, it is the responsibility of every practitioner to consult appropriate information sources to ascertain correct dosages for each clinical situation, especially for new or unfamiliar drugs and procedures. The authors, editors, publisher, and the Department of Defense cannot be held responsible for any errors found in this book.

Use of Trade or Brand Names: Use of trade or brand names in this publication is for illustrative purposes only and does not imply endorsement by the Department of Defense.

Neutral Language: Unless this publication states otherwise, masculine nouns and pronouns do not refer exclusively to men.

The opinions or assertions contained herein are the personal views of the authors and are not to be construed as doctrine of the Department of the Army or the Department of Defense. For comments or suggestions on additional contents in forthcoming editions, please contact the publisher (www.cs.amedd.army.mil/borden).

Published by the Office of The Surgeon General
Borden Institute
Fort Sam Houston, Texas

Contents

US Army Medical Research Institute of Chemical Defense

Editors

Colonel (Ret) Gary Hurst, Medical Corps, US Army
Lieutenant Colonel John Stich, AN, US Army
Lieutenant Colonel (Ret) Tim Byrne, Medical Corps, US Air Force
Colonel Martha K. Lenhart, Medical Corps, US Army
Daniel Boehm
Laukton Rimpel
Staff Sergeant Gary Hall, US Army

Acknowledgements

Colonel James Madsen, Medical Corps, US Army

Introduction

Purpose

Poisoning by (ie, exposure to) toxic chemicals, a process also called intoxication, has been an important medical issue for centuries. A particularly frightening type of poisoning is the generation of mass casualties on the battlefield by the use of either chemicals developed specifically for that purpose or chemicals produced for industry and coopted for battlefield use. These agents can also produce civilian casualties during warfare and, when used by terrorists, cause both military and civilian casualties in settings remote from a defined battlefield.

Military healthcare providers have a responsibility to recognize and manage chemical casualties whatever the setting. This is primarily because military healthcare providers will likely be the first medical personnel to receive exposed service members. Secondly, because of the preeminence of the US military medical establishment in research, response, and training in chemical warfare agents, military medical personnel must be able to respond to chemical exposures at US stockpile sites of chemical warfare agents and provide expert consultation to their civilian counterparts in the event of a terrorist attack involving these agents. Knowledge of the medical aspects of the prevention, preparedness, response, and recovery phases of any military or civilian event involving chemical exposure is expected of every military medical care provider.

This handbook has been produced to help address the need for first provider training. Its primary use is as an adjunct, together with a companion biological agent handbook, to the Medical Management of Chemical and Biological Casualties (MCBC) course offered jointly by the US Army Medical Research Institute of Chemical Defense (USAMRICD) and the US Army Medical Research Institute of Infectious Disease. It is intended not to replace the hands-on training afforded by this course, but to provide an additional resource for MCBC students both during the course and after its completion.

The treatment protocols and drug dosages described in this handbook are not to be construed as replacements for sound clinical judgment. Please utilize the Internet site of USAMRICD's Chemical Casualty Care Division for the latest available resources: http://ccc.apgea.army.mil.

Nine appendices at the end of this handbook illustrate and summarize the major concepts of the publication. Review cards for each type of agent presented can be found in the back of the handbook.

Chemical Agents: General Concepts and Terminology

To paraphrase Paracelsus, any substance delivered in excess can act as a poison; it is the dose that makes the poison. Even oxygen can be toxic to the central nervous system at high partial pressures. Nevertheless, the term *poison* traditionally refers to chemicals that are sufficiently potent to induce poisoning in relatively low doses. The terms *toxic chemical, chemical agent,* and *chemical warfare agent* are often defined in different ways, and their use in this handbook needs to be clarified at the outset, along with the use of related terms.

The Chemical Warfare Convention (CWC) is an arms control treaty that outlaws the production, stockpiling, and use of chemical weapons and their precursors. The CWC defines a *toxic chemical* as "any chemical which through its chemical action on life processes can cause death, temporary incapacitation or permanent harm to humans or animals"; specifies that this definition includes "all such chemicals, regardless of their origin or their method of production"; and specifically includes toxins such as ricin and saxitoxin. Toxic chemicals can also be produced from precursors that include binary or multicomponent chemical systems. Not all chemical warfare agent precursors are listed under the CWC.

The US Army defines *chemical warfare agents* (often called simply *chemical agents*) as toxic substances developed for military use to produce death, serious injury, or incapacitation through their toxicological effects on exposed humans or animals. The Army officially excludes from this definition three broad categories of chemicals: (1) riot-control agents, (2) herbicides, and (3) smoke and flame materials.

Toxic industrial materials, or TIMs, are industry-associated materials with harmful effects on humans; they can be subdivided into *toxic industrial biologicals*, or TIBs; *toxic industrial chemicals*, or TICs; and *toxic industrial radiologicals*, or TIRs. The North Atlantic Treaty Organization (NATO) has a more restricted definition for *toxic industrial chemical* as a chemical that (1) is more toxic than ammonia and (2) is produced in quantities greater than 30 tons per year at a given production facility. However, TICs are also commonly defined as any industrially manufactured chemicals that could be used to produce mass casualties.

Toxicant is a general synonym for *poison* and can be used interchangeably with the latter term. *Toxin* is also commonly used as a synonym for poison, but in discussions of chemical and biological agents is best defined in its more restricted sense as a toxic chemical synthesized by a living organism. Toxins have characteristics of both chemical and biological agents and are increasingly being separately classified as *mid-spectrum agents*, which include not only toxins but also bioregulators (small molecules with regulatory functions in the body in physiological doses but with toxic effects in larger doses), synthetic viruses, and genocidal weapons.

Chemical, biological, and mid-spectrum agents are often referred to as *weapons of mass destruction*, or WMDs, and the official military definition of WMD includes these three kinds of agents. However, in the strict sense of the term, weapons of mass destruction are weapons capable of causing extensive damage to physical structures, such as buildings, and include high explosives and nuclear and thermonuclear bombs. Chemical agents, biological agents, toxins, and point sources of radiation may cause mass casualties while leaving structures intact; a better term for these kinds of weapons is *mass-casualty weapons*, or MCWs. *Unconventional weapons* is a term used to refer to chemical agents, biological agents, toxins, nuclear and thermonuclear bombs, radiological dispersal devices (or RDDs, also called "dirty bombs"), and point sources of radiation used as weapons.

The list of chemical warfare agents officially designated as such by the US military includes those chemicals that are intended to cause death or serious injury and also those intended to cause incapacitation, that is, temporary inability to perform one's military duties. The former are called *toxic agents* and include (1) lung-damaging agents (also called pulmonary or choking agents); (2) "blood" agents (specifically, cyanide compounds); (3) vesicants (blistering agents); and (4) nerve agents. Those designed to produce only temporary incapacitation are referred to as *incapacitating agents*. This handbook will address each of these groupings of "official" chemical warfare agents as well as riot-control agents, which are technically not chemical warfare agents according to the US military definition, but are widely used in law enforcement for mass incapacitation.

Chemical agents may have chemical names as well as common names. Chemical agents developed for military use may also have a NATO code. The NATO code is a one- to three-letter designation assigned after World War II to provide standard recognizable shorthand identification. For example, the chemical compound O-isopropyl methylphosphonofluoridate has the common name sarin and the NATO code GB. This handbook will use NATO codes as well as common names for chemical agents.

Physical Forms of Chemical Agents

Chemical agents, like all other substances, may exist as solids, liquids, or gases, depending on temperature and pressure. Except for riot-control agents and the incapacitating agent BZ, which are solids at usually encountered temperatures and pressures, chemical agents in munitions are liquids. Following detonation of the munitions container, the agent is primarily dispersed as liquid or as an *aerosol*, defined as a collection of very small solid particles or liquid droplets suspended in a gas (in this case, in the explosive gases and the atmosphere). Thus, "tear gas," a riot-control agent, is not really a gas at all, but rather an aerosolized solid. Likewise, mustard "gas" and nerve "gas" do not become true gases even at the boiling point of water (212°F / 100°C at sea level).

Certain chemical agents, such as hydrogen cyanide, chlorine, and phosgene, may be gases when encountered during warm months of the year at sea level. The nerve agents and mustard are liquids under these conditions, but they are to a certain extent volatile as temperature rises; that is, they volatilize or evaporate, just as water or gasoline does, to form an often invisible *vapor*. A vapor is the gaseous form of a substance that is normally a liquid at usual environmental temperatures. Another way to conceptualize a vapor is as the gaseous form of a substance at a temperature lower than the boiling point of that substance at a given pressure. Liquid water, for example, becomes a gas (steam) when heated to its boiling point at a given pressure, but below that temperature, it slowly evaporates to form water vapor, which is invisible. Visible water clouds (including "clouds of steam") are composed neither of water vapor nor water gas (steam), but rather are suspensions of minute water droplets (ie, an aerosol).

The tendency of a chemical agent to evaporate depends not only on its chemical composition and on the temperature and air pressure, but also on such variables as wind velocity and the nature of the underlying surface the agent is in contact with. Just as water evaporates less quickly than gasoline but more quickly than motor oil at a given temperature, pure mustard is less volatile than the nerve agent GB but more volatile than the nerve agent VX. However, all of these agents evaporate more readily when the temperature rises, when a strong wind is blowing, or when they are resting on glass rather than on, for example, porous fabric.

Volatility is thus inversely related to persistence, because the more volatile a substance is, the more quickly it evaporates and the less it tends to stay or persist as a liquid and contaminate terrain and materiel. The liquid hazard of a persistent agent is often more significant than the danger created by the relatively small amounts of vapor it may generate. The converse is true of nonpersistent agents, which may pose a serious vapor hazard but which also evaporate quickly enough not to create a liquid hazard for an extended time. The generally accepted division between persistent and nonpersistent agents is 24 hours, meaning that a persistent agent will constitute a liquid hazard and contaminate surfaces for 24 hours or longer. Such agents (mustard and VX) are thus suitable for contaminating and denying terrain and materiel to the enemy. Nonpersistent agents, such as GB and cyanide, find tactical employment in the direct line of assault into enemy territory since they will have evaporated within a day and will no longer contaminate surfaces. These generalizations are obviously subject to the modifying factors of temperature, environmental factors such as wind, and surface characteristics.

Exposure, Absorption, and Toxicity of Chemical Agents

Toxicologically speaking, exposure means contact of a poison with an epithelial surface (such as the skin, respiratory epithelium, eyes, or gastrointestinal mucosa) and is an external dose. Penetration of an epithelial barrier is called absorption and results in an absorbed dose, or internal dose. An absorbed agent may exert local effects at or near the site of exposure and absorption or systemic effects following distribution in the circulation to sites remote from the exposure site (eg, as in liquid nerve agents absorbed through the skin). Biological effects occur following exposure to chemical agents dispersed as solids, liquids, gases, aerosols, or vapors. Eye or skin injury may follow direct exposure to the suspended solid particles of aerosolized riot-control agents, and inhalation of these agents brings the aerosolized solid in contact with the epithelium of the respiratory tree. Nevertheless, systemic effects from exposure to riot-control agents are rare. Contact of the eyes, or more likely the skin, with liquid nerve or vesicant agents may produce local effects or lead to absorption and systemic effects.

Liquid exposure is the most important hazard associated with persistent agents. Healthcare providers managing liquid exposure must properly wear chemical protective clothing. At low temperatures, hydrogen cyanide (AC), cyanogen chloride (CK), and phosgene (CG) exist as liquids. However, because of their high volatility (low persistence), they seldom present a significant liquid hazard unless the area of exposure is large or evaporation is impeded when liquid agent is trapped in saturated, porous clothing. Penetration of fragments or clothing contaminated with liquid chemical agent of any type may also lead to intramuscular or intravenous exposure and subsequent systemic effects.

Chemical agents in the form of aerosolized liquid droplets, vapor, or gas may come into direct contact with the eyes, skin, or (through inhalation) the pulmonary compartments. Local damage is possible at any of these sites, but systemic absorption through dry, intact skin is usually less important than with the other routes. Vapor or gas exposure to the eyes, and especially the respiratory tree, is the most important hazard associated with nonpersistent agents; to prevent such exposure, a mask that provides both ocular and inhalation protection must be properly worn.

Specialized terms refer to the amount of chemical agent encountered during an exposure. The effective dose, denoted by ED_{50}, and the incapacitating dose, denoted by ID_{50}, refer to the quantities (usually measured as the weight in µg, mg, or g) of liquid agent that will predictably cause effects (E) or incapacitation (I) in 50% of a given group. Similarly, the lethal dose, denoted by LD_{50}, refers to the quantity (weight) of liquid agent that will kill 50% of a group. Note that the *lower* the LD_{50}, the *less* agent is required and thus the *more potent* the agent is. Because of differences in absorption, the ED_{50} and LD_{50} values for a given agent are site-specific; for example, the LD_{50} for mustard absorbed through dry, unabraded skin is much higher than the LD_{50} for mustard absorbed through the eye.

Comparison of the amounts of chemical agent encountered as aerosol, vapor, or gas requires use of the concentration-time product, or Ct, which refers to the agent concentration (usually in mg/m^3) multiplied by the time (usually in minutes) of exposure. For example, exposure to a concentration of 4 mg/m^3 of agent vapor for 10 minutes results in a Ct of 40 $mg{\cdot}min/m^3$. Exposure to 8 mg/m^3 for 5 minutes results in the same Ct (40 $mg{\bullet}min/m^3$). For almost any given agent (with the notable exception of cyanide, which will be discussed in a separate chapter), the Ct associated with a biological effect is relatively constant even though the concentration and time components may vary within certain limits (Haber's law). Therefore, a 10-minute exposure to 4 mg/m^3 of agent causes the same effects as a 5-minute exposure to 8 mg/m^3 or to a 1-minute exposure to 40 mg/m^3. The ECt_{50}, ICt_{50}, and LCt_{50} correspond for vapor or gas exposures to the ED_{50}, ID_{50}, and LD_{50}, respectively, for liquid exposure and are likewise site-specific. However, the Ct does not take into account variables such as respiratory rate and depth and is therefore not an exact measure of inhalation exposure.

General Principles of Chemical Casualty Care

Chemical casualties must be recognized and appropriately managed. Management includes *triage, medical treatment, decontamination* (if liquid contamination is present), and *disposition,* which may include evacuation and eventual return to duty.

Casualty Recognition

Recognition of a chemical casualty is heavily dependent upon recognition and differential diagnosis of *toxidromes,* that is, constellations of symptoms and signs that characterize exposure to a specific agent, as well as intelligence reports and detection equipment. This handbook will present distinct toxidromes characteristic of exposure to central-compartment lung-damaging agents, peripheral-compartment lung-damaging agents, cyanide compounds, sulfur mustard, lewisite, phosgene oxime, nerve agents, anticholinergic incapacitating agents, "traditional" riot-control agents, and vomiting agents (a subset of riot-control agents). It is important to recognize these toxidromes and also to recognize other conditions that could mimic them.

Chemical agent casualties may be exposed to more than one agent and may also have other diagnoses, such as concomitant exposure to other kinds of mass-casualty agents, preexisting medical or surgical conditions, or trauma. It is just as important to view the casualty, and the situation, as a whole as it is to identify chemical exposure. The best way to accomplish this is to consider the triad of *agent, environment,* and *host*. Specifically, the astute clinician will think of (1) the agent; (2) the forms or states of the agent in the environment; (3) the passage of agent from the environment to the host, that is, the route or routes of entry; (4) whether exposure and absorption by the host are producing only local effects (restricted to the site of exposure) or are also generating systemic effects (effects remote from the site of exposure); (5) the severity of exposure and of effects; (6) the time course of effects; (7) other possible differential diagnoses and concomitant diagnoses; and (8) any possible interaction or synergism among coexisting diagnoses. Healthcare providers engaged in treatment have a tendency to focus on the chemical exposure, sometimes to the neglect of other life-threatening conditions.

Casualty Management

Once a chemical casualty has been recognized, appropriate management must begin. *Triage* is the process of sorting casualties for medical treatment when not all casualties can receive care simultaneously. It is in some ways both an assessment step and a management step and can act as a bridge between initial assessment and management. The triage categories used by the US military are (1) *immediate* (those who are in danger of losing their lives unless action is taken within a few minutes); (2) *delayed* (those who require significant medical intervention but who can tolerate a longer delay in treatment); (3) *minimal* (casualties who have minor injuries, illnesses, or intoxications, often amenable to self or buddy care); and (4) *expectant* (those who are gravely ill and who cannot be treated with available resources without causing the death, by misallocation of resources, of other casualties). In this handbook, triage for specific chemical agents will be addressed within the chapter devoted to that agent.

Initial management for severely affected chemical casualties (especially those who are triaged as immediate) can be summarized as an application of the ABCDDs: **A**irway, **B**reathing, **C**irculation, immediate **D**econtamination, and **D**rugs (ie, specific antidotes). These interventions will be described in specific agent chapters and also in the sections on decontamination and casualty management in a contaminated area. It is important to note that the ABCDDs might have to be applied nonsequentially, for example, during a nerve agent poisoning, atropine may have to be administered to ease airway restriction first. Immediate decontamination may mitigate the effects of the agent.

Chapter 1

LUNG-DAMAGING AGENTS: TOXIC INDUSTRIAL CHEMICALS

Summary

NATO Codes: CG, Cl

Signs and Symptoms: Central effects: eye and airway irritation, dyspnea; peripheral effects: chest tightness and *delayed* pulmonary edema.

Field Detection: Joint Chemical Agent Detector (JCAD). The M18A2 Chemical Agent Detector Kit and the M93 series Fox Reconnaissance System will detect small concentrations of CG; however, they will not detect Cl.

Decontamination: *Vapor:* fresh air; *liquid:* copious water irrigation.

Management: Termination of exposure, ABCs of resuscitation (airway, breathing, circulation), enforced rest and observation, oxygen with or without positive airway pressure for signs of respiratory distress, other supportive therapy as needed.

Overview

Over 1,800 toxic industrial chemicals (TICs) are used in industry, stored at industrial sites, and transported on the world's road and rail systems. Some of these chemicals were deployed as chemical warfare agents during the First World War, killing and injuring thousands, and can have the same deadly consequences today if released during an accident or through terrorist sabotage. Death from exposure to TICs is more frequent when they are inhaled. Inhaling a TIC in the form of a gas, vapor (gas coming from a liquid), or aerosol (liquid or solid particles suspended in a gas) can cause a sudden closure of the larynx (laryngospasm), causing the victim to choke and collapse. TICs can also cause damage to the tissues of the upper airways, resulting in swelling, scarring, and airway narrowing, which can restrict breathing. TICs can damage lung tissues, allowing body plasma and other fluids to leak into the lung air sacs (alveoli), causing pulmonary edema and death from asphyxiation.

Lung-damaging TICs are typically heavier than air and hang close to the ground when released. They tend to evaporate and disperse very quickly, depending on temperature and wind conditions (Table 1-1). If the TIC is in liquid form at room temperature, it will tend to give off a vapor. Vapors can become trapped in clothing fibers and "off-gas" to affect anyone nearby with no respiratory protection. Although skin decontamination after vapor exposure is not a high priority, clothing should be removed and the underlying skin decontaminated with soap and water.

Table 1-1. Physiochemical Characteristics of Toxic Industrial Chemicals

Agent	Molecular Weight	Boiling Point	Freezing Point	Distinctive Odor
Phosgene (CG)	99	7.6°C	−128°C	Newly mown hay
Hydrogen chloride (HCl)	36.46	−85°C	−114°C	Pungent
Ammonia	17.03	−33.4°C	−77.7°C	Sharp, intensely irritating
Perfluoroisobutylene	Polymer	214°C −217°C	257°C −263°C	None
Oxides of nitrogen (NOx)	28.1	−196°C	−210°C	Irritating
White phosphorus smoke	123.895	280°C	44.1°C	Garlic-like

Exposure to TIC lung-damaging agents can occur on and off the battlefield. The care provider must know how to identify the signs and symptoms and provide appropriate life-saving support to those exposed to these agents.

Understanding the Respiratory System

The respiratory system can be divided into two compartments, the central airway and the peripheral airway (Figure 1-1). Understanding these compartments can greatly simplify the treatment problem-solving process.

The *central airway compartment* includes the nasopharynx (nose), oropharynx (mouth), larynx (vocal cords), and the trachea and bronchi (airway from the throat into the lungs). Tissues in this area are very moist and thin and can be damaged by TICs.

The *peripheral lung compartment* includes the lung sacs

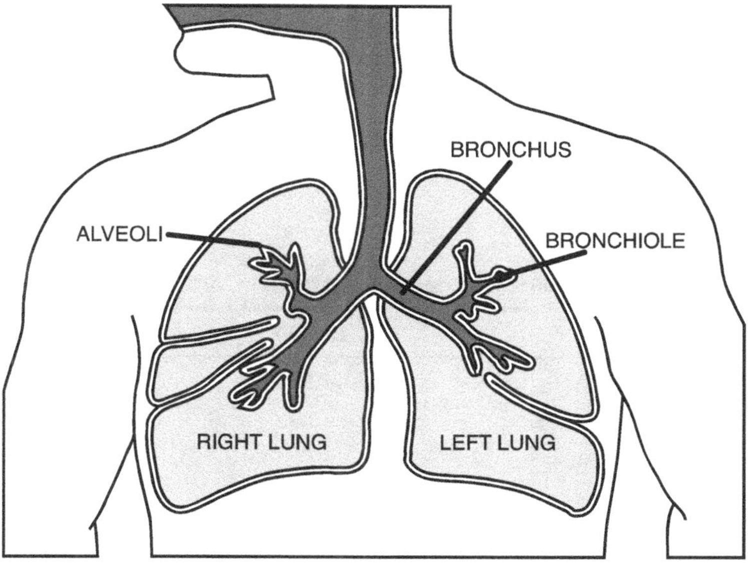

Figure 1-1. Central airway (dark gray) and peripheral airway (light gray).

(alveoli) distributed throughout the lung tissue. During normal respiration, inhaled gasses fill the alveoli and then move slowly through their walls. The gasses then move through the thin walls of the blood vessels (capillaries) surrounding the alveoli and into the blood. TICs can damage the walls of alveoli and the capillaries surrounding them, allowing blood plasma and cells to leak into the air space of the alveoli.

Lung-Damaging Agents

TICs are numerous. Those that pose a frequent threat to the service members in the field are listed below. Though the list is not complete, casualties from other lung-damaging agents are managed the same way as these examples. In low doses, highly reactive TICs have a greater effect on the central airway; other TICs act on both airways; and still others that are not as reactive in the central airway travel deeper into the respiratory tract and destroy alveoli tissues in the peripheral airways (Table 1-2). Any TIC inhaled in large doses will cause damage to both central and peripheral airways.

Centrally Acting TICS

Ammonia is highly caustic and reactive gas used for cleaning, industrial refrigeration, and numerous other legitimate industrial

Table 1-2. Toxic Industrial Chemicals Compartment of Action

Agent	Central	Peripheral
Phosgene (CG)	Large dose	Yes
Oxides of nitrogen (NOx)	Large dose	Yes
HC smoke	Large dose	Yes
Ammonia	Yes	Large dose
Chloride (Cl)	Yes	Yes
Perfluoroisobutylene	Large dose	Yes

processes, as well as for processing some illicit drugs. It is a good example of a TIC that, in low doses, is primarily centrally acting. It rapidly forms a strong base (alkali) when it contacts the moist tissues of the central airway compartment. The alkali burns and destroys the tissues it contacts. The victim may suddenly go into laryngospasm and collapse. The tissues of the compartment become swollen. Scar tissue may form along the airway. Damaged tissue in the airway may die and slough off, obstructing the airway.

Sulfur mustard (HD) is an example of a chemical agent produced solely for warfare that acts on the central airway compartment when inhaled. HD will cause tissue to slough off in large sheets, known as pseudomembranes, which block the airway. The various resulting degrees of airway obstruction cause hoarseness or wheezing, or prevent casualties from breathing, sneezing, or coughing.

Peripherally Acting TICs

Phosgene (CG) is a major industrial chemical used in many manufacturing processes. More importantly, it is released from heating or burning many common chemicals or solvents. Carbon tetrachloride, perchloroethylene (a degreasing compound), methylene chloride (used in paint removal), and many other compounds break down to phosgene with flame or heat. Also, common substances such as foam plastics release phosgene when they burn. A soldier presenting with shortness of breath in the absence of a chemical attack or other obvious cause should be questioned carefully about whether he or she has been near any burning substances or chemical vapors that were near flame or other hot materials (eg, a heater with open coils).

Perfluoroisobutylene (PFIB) is given off when Teflon (DuPont, Wilmington, DE) burns at high temperatures, such as in a vehicle fire. Teflon is used to line the interior of many military vehicles, particularly armored vehicles and aircraft. Closed-space fires in these vehicles release PFIB. Survivors of vehicle fires who are short of breath should be questioned about their exposure to the smoke.

Oxides of nitrogen (NOx) are components of photochemical smog that can be produced by the burning of gunpowder or industrial waste. These substances can build up to high concentrations where artillery is fired and there is inadequate ventilation. Soldiers who become short of breath after heavy firing should be suspected of exposure to this lung-damaging agent.

HC smoke is a mixture of equal amounts of hexachloroethane, zinc oxide, and approximately 7% grained aluminum or aluminum powder used in the military for obscuration. The zinc oxide can cause lung damage if inhaled in toxic amounts. Appropriate precautions, such as wearing protective masks, must be taken when HC smoke is used.

TICs That Act Both Centrally and Peripherally

Chlorine (Cl) is a good example of a combination agent, one that acts on both airway compartments in low doses. It is widely used in industry for manufacturing plastics and lubricants and purifying water. It was the first chemical agent used effectively on the First World War battlefield against unprotected military troops, but its effectiveness as a weapon was greatly reduced once protective masks became widely available to soldiers. Chlorine turns to hydrochloric acid when it contacts the moisture of the airway; it then causes chemical burns to the tissue. It produces signs and symptoms seen with exposure to both central and peripherally acting agents. Its action serves as a reminder that although central compartment damage may seem like the primary concern in some patients (eg, they are coughing and wheezing), the medic must always treat casualties as if they could develop peripheral compartment symptoms, and take seriously any patient complaints about feeling chest tightness or having breathing difficulty.

Detection

Chlorine and ammonia have their own distinctive odors. Phosgene smells like newly cut grass, newly mown hay, or green corn. It is important to remember that odor is not a reliable detection method. Smelling the gas exposes the individual to potentially toxic inhalation effects. There are no specific field detection devices for these compounds.

Protection

The military protective mask, if fitted with a C2A1 filter canister, or the Joint Service General Purpose Mask with M61 filters will protect against Cl, CG, PFIB, NOx, and HC smoke in the open battlefield. Specific filters, or the use of a self-contained breathing apparatus, are mandated for other TICs, such as ammonia. Masks do not protect against carbon dioxide, and they are not be effective in environments where the TIC displaces oxygen, creating a low oxygen environment (at or below 19.5% fraction of expired oxygen [FiO_2]). Masks should only be used in these environments for escape purposes. A self-contained breathing apparatus is recommended.

Toxicity

The median lethal concentration (LCt_{50}) of phosgene is approximately half the LCt_{50} of chlorine. Since only half as much phosgene is required to kill half of an exposed group, phosgene is thus twice as potent as chlorine. PFIB is ten times more toxic than phosgene. Table 1-3 lists the Occupational Safety and Health Administration standards for exposure limits in parts per million.

Table 1-3. Occupational Safety and Health Administration Standards for Toxic Industrial Chemical Exposure Limits

Agent	Concentrated Exposure Limits (ppm)
Phosgene (CG)	0.1
Chloride (Cl)	5
Ammonia	50
Perfluoroisobutylene	0.01
Oxides of nitrogen (NOx)	25
White phosphorus smoke	1

Toxicodynamics: Mechanisms of Action

Central compartment. Centrally acting TICs such as ammonia and HD form strong acids or bases (alkali) when in contact with the water in the central airway tissues, and then destroy these tissues. Damaged tissues will swell and can slough into the airway and restrict breathing.

Peripheral compartment. Phosgene is the most studied peripheral compartment agent. It causes pulmonary edema, which is life threatening. Less is known about the other compounds; however, they are believed to be very similar.

Phosgene causes effects in the lung by inhalation only. It does not affect the lung when absorbed through the skin, injected, or orally ingested. When inhaled, phosgene travels to the very end of the smallest airways, the bronchioles, and causes damage to these airways. Additionally, it damages the thin membrane that separates the smallest blood vessels (the capillaries) and the air sacs (the alveoli) by reacting with the proteins and enzymes in the membranes. These membranes usually separate the blood in the capillaries from the air in the alveoli, but when the membranes are damaged, they cannot perform this function. Blood, or at least plasma (the liquid part of the blood), can leak through the damaged membrane into the alveoli. When plasma leaks into the alveoli, the air sacs become full of fluid, and air cannot enter them. Therefore, exchange of oxygen from the air into the blood is hindered, and the casualty suffers oxygen deprivation. The extent of oxygen deprivation depends on the extent of the phosgene exposure and the number of alveoli filled with plasma. The mechanism is similar to what happens with drowning, in that the alveoli fill up with fluid; however, in this instance, it is fluid from the blood, not from an external source. For this reason, phosgene poisoning is sometimes referred to as "dry land drowning."

Clinical Effects

Centrally acting agents. Immediately or shortly after exposure to these gasses or vapors, the casualty can develop laryngospasm, though not in all exposures. As the airways become irritated and damaged, the individual will sneeze and experience pain in the nose (nasopharynx inflammation) and may develop painful swallowing (oropharynx inflammation); hoarseness, a feeling of choking, and noise with exhalation (larynx inflammation); and pain in the chest, coughing, and wheezing during breathing (trachea and bronchi inflammation). If the exposure has been enough to cause the TIC to reach the peripheral compartment, peripheral effects can follow. Scarring of the central airway can create permanent airway narrowing depending on the agent involved and the dose received.

Peripherally acting agents. The *major effects* from phosgene and other peripherally acting agents *do not occur until hours after exposure.* Immediately after exposure to these agents, the casualty will typically have an asymptomatic period of 30 minutes to 72 hours, but in most significant exposures the latent period is less than 24 hours. The duration and concentration of the exposure will determine the time to symptom onset. The casualty may notice irritation of the eyes, nose, and throat, but more commonly there are no effects during or immediately after exposure. HD signs are also delayed, but the damage is more in the central compartment.

The casualty with peripheral compartment damage who is developing pulmonary edema will notice shortness of breath (dyspnea) between 2 and 24 hours after exposure. Initially, this may be mild, and the eventual severity of the dyspnea depends on the amount of exposure. As the damage progresses, the dyspnea becomes more severe, and soon a cough develops. If the damage is severe, the casualty begins coughing up clear, foamy sputum, the plasma that has leaked into the alveoli.

Casualties with a very mild exposure to phosgene (or another of these compounds) will develop dyspnea 6 to 24 hours after exposure. They will notice it first after heavy exertion; however, later they become short of breath after any activity. With proper care, these casualties do well and recover completely.

A casualty with a severe exposure to phosgene (or another of these compounds) will notice shortness of breath within 4 to 6 hours after exposure. Increased difficulty breathing, even at rest, will occur, and even with intensive pulmonary care, the casualty may not survive.

The average exposure to a lung-damaging agent will fall between these two extreme cases. When the onset of dyspnea is greater than 6 hours after exposure, there may be progression to dyspnea at rest. However, with good pulmonary care beginning early after the onset of effects, the individual should recover completely.

Differential Diagnosis

Many TICs can be distinguished by their odor; they generally irritate the mucous membranes and can lead to dyspnea and pulmonary edema of delayed onset. In contrast, riot-control agents produce a burning sensation, predominantly in the eyes and upper airways, that is typically more intense than that caused by TICs and is unaccompanied by their distinctive odors. Nerve agents induce the production of watery secretions as well as respiratory distress; however, their other characteristic effects distinguish nerve agent toxicity from TIC inhalation injury.

The respiratory toxicity associated with vesicants is usually delayed but predominantly affects the central, rather than the peripheral, compartment. Vesicant inhalation severe enough to cause dyspnea typically causes signs of airway necrosis, often with pseudomembrane formation and partial or complete upper airway obstruction. Finally, pulmonary parenchymal damage following vesicant exposure usually manifests itself as hemorrhage rather than pulmonary edema.

Laboratory Findings

No commonly available laboratory tests exist for the specific identification or quantification of exposure to lung-damaging agents. However, an increase in the hematocrit may reflect the hemoconcentration induced by transudation of fluid into the pulmonary parenchyma from peripherally acting agents. Arterial blood gases may show a low PaO_2 or $PaCO_2$, which is an early, nonspecific warning of increased interstitial fluid in the lung.

Decreased lung compliance and carbon monoxide diffusing capacity are particularly sensitive indicators of interstitial fluid volume in the lung, but these are complex tests for hospital use only.

With peripherally acting agents, early findings on chest x-ray are hyperinflation, followed later by pulmonary edema without cardiovascular changes of redistribution or cardiomegaly. Ventilation profusion ratio (V/Q) scanning is very sensitive but is nonspecific and for hospital use only.

Medical Management

1. *Terminate exposure* as a vital first measure. This may be accomplished by physically removing casualties from the contaminated environment or by isolating them from surrounding contamination by supplying a properly fitting mask. Decontamination of any liquid agent on skin, and removal of clothing if vapors are trapped there, fully terminates exposure from that source.
2. *Execute the ABCs* (airway, breathing, circulation) of resuscitation as required. Establishing an airway is especially crucial in a patient exhibiting hoarseness or stridor; such individuals may face impending laryngeal spasm and require intubation. Establishing a clear airway also aids in interpreting auscultatory findings. Steps to minimize the work of breathing must be taken. Because of the always present danger of hypotension induced by pulmonary edema or positive airway pressure, accurate determination of the casualty's circulatory status is vital not just initially but also at regularly repeated intervals and whenever indicated by the clinical situation.
3. *Enforce rest.* Even minimal physical exertion may shorten the clinical latent period and increase the severity of respiratory symptoms and signs in a lung-damaging agent casualty. Physical activity in a symptomatic patient may precipitate acute clinical deterioration and even death. Strict limitation of activity (ie, forced bed rest) and litter evacuation are mandatory for patients suspected of having inhaled any of the edematogenic agents. This is true whether or not the patient has respiratory symptoms and whether or not objective evidence of pulmonary edema is present.
4. *Prepare to manage airway secretions and prevent/treat bronchospasm.* Unless superinfection is present, secretions in the airways

of lung-damaging agent casualties are usually copious and watery. They may serve as an index to the degree of pulmonary edema and do not require specific therapy apart from suctioning and drainage. Antibiotics should be reserved for those patients with an infectious process documented by sputum Gram staining and culture. Bronchospasm may occur in individuals with reactive airways, and these patients should receive theophylline or beta-adrenergic bronchodilators.

Steroid therapy is also indicated for bronchospasm as long as parenteral administration is chosen over topical therapy, which may result in inadequate distribution to damaged airways. Methylprednisolone, 700 to 1,000 mg, or its equivalent, may be given intravenously in divided doses during the first day and then tapered off during the duration of the clinical illness. Increased susceptibility to bacterial infection during steroid therapy mandates careful surveillance of the patient. There is some support in the literature for steroid use in those exposed to HC smoke (zinc/zinc oxide) and NOx, as these agents are theorized to reduce autoimmune reactions that can foster scar development and subsequent bronchiolitis obliterans. The literature does not give strong support for the use of steroids in the treatment of other toxic inhalants. Thus, steroids are not recommended in individuals without evidence of overt or latent reactive airway disease.

5. *Prevent and treat hypoxia.* Oxygen therapy is definitely indicated and may require supplemental positive airway pressure administered via one of several available devices for generating intermittent or continuous positive pressure. Intubation, with or without ventilatory assistance, may be required, and positive pressure may need to be applied during at least the end-expiratory phase of the ventilator cycle.
6. *Prevent and treat pulmonary edema.* Positive airway pressure provides some control over the clinical complications of pulmonary edema. Early use of a positive pressure mask may be beneficial. Positive airway pressure may exacerbate hypotension by decreasing thoracic venous return, necessitating intravenous fluid administration.
7. *Prevent and treat hypotension.* Sequestration of plasma-derived

fluid in the lungs may cause hypotension that may be exacerbated by positive airway pressure. Urgent intravenous administration of either crystalloid or colloid (in this situation) both appear equally effective. The use of vasopressors is a temporary measure until fluids can be replaced.

Triage

Patients seen within 12 hours of exposure. A patient with pulmonary edema only is classified *immediate* if intensive pulmonary care is immediately available. In general, a shorter latent period portends a more serious illness. A *delayed* patient is dyspneic without objective signs and should be observed closely and retriaged hourly. An asymptomatic patient with known exposure should be classified *minimal* and observed and retriaged every 2 hours. If this patient remains asymptomatic 24 hours after exposure, he or she should be discharged. If exposure is in doubt and the patient remains asymptomatic 12 hours following putative exposure, consider discharge. An *expectant* patient presents with pulmonary edema, cyanosis, and hypotension. A casualty who presents with these signs within 6 hours of exposure generally will not survive; a casualty with the onset of these signs 6 hours or longer after exposure may survive with immediate, intensive medical care. If ventilatory support is not available but adequate evacuation assets are, these patients should have priority for urgent evacuation to a facility with adequate ventilatory resources.

Patients seen more than 12 hours after exposure. A patient with pulmonary edema is classified *immediate* provided he or she will receive intensive care within several hours. If cyanosis and hypotension are also present, triage the patient as *expectant*. A *delayed* patient is dyspneic and should be observed closely and retriaged every 2 hours. If the patient is recovering, discharge him or her 24 hours after exposure. An asymptomatic patient or patient with resolving dyspnea is classified *minimal*. If the patient is asymptomatic 24 hours after exposure, he or she should be discharged. A patient with persistent hypotension despite intensive medical care is *expectant*.

Return to Duty

If the patient has only eye or upper airway irritation and is asymptomatic with normal physical examination 12 hours after exposure, he or she may be returned to duty. If the patient's original complaint was dyspnea only, yet physical examination, chest x-ray, and arterial blood gases are all normal at 24 hours, he or she may be returned to duty. If the patient presented initially with symptoms *and* an abnormal physical examination, chest x-ray, or arterial blood gas, he or she requires close supervision but can be returned to duty at 48 hours if physical examination, chest x-ray, and arterial blood gases are all normal at that time.

Chapter 2

CYANIDE

Summary

NATO Codes: AC, CK

Signs and Symptoms: Few; seizures, respiratory and cardiac arrest after exposure to high concentrations.

Field Detection: The Joint Chemical Agent Detector (JCAD), M256A1 Chemical Agent Detector Kit, M18A2 Chemical Agent Detector Kit, and M90 Chemical Warfare Agent Detector detect hydrogen cyanide (AC) as vapor or gas in the air, and the M272 Chemical Agent Water Testing Kit detects AC in water.

Decontamination: Skin decontamination is usually not necessary because the agents are highly volatile. Wet, contaminated clothing should be removed and the underlying skin decontaminated with water or other standard decontaminants to prevent off-gassing as a hazard.

Management: Antidote: intravenous (IV) sodium nitrite, inhalational amyl nitrite, and sodium thiosulfate. *Supportive:* oxygen, correct acidosis.

Overview

Cyanide is a rapidly acting, lethal agent that is limited in its military usefulness by its high median lethal concentration (LCt_{50}) and high volatility. Death occurs about 8 minutes after inhalation of a high concentration. Amyl nitrite, sodium nitrite,and sodium thiosulfate are effective antidotes. An alternative antidote, hydroxocobalamin, is also effective. With any antidote, 100% oxygen has been empirically shown to be beneficial.

History and Military Relevance

The French used cyanide in World War I without notable military success, possibly because of the insufficient amounts delivered and the nature of the chemical. In Germany, Nazis used cyanide in the extermination of death camp prisoners. Zyklon B, a cyanide-based pesticide, was used in enclosed chambers. Nazi leaders used cyanide to commit suicide. The United States maintained a small number of cyanide munitions during World War II. Japan allegedly used cyanide against China before and during World War II, and Iraq may have used cyanide against the Kurds in the 1980s. In 1978 the Jim Jones cult staged a mass suicide in Guyana, where over 900 followers drank a cyanide- laced beverage. In 1982 cyanide contamination of Tylenol (McNEIL-PPC, Inc; Fort Washington, PA) led to the production of tamper-proof bottle caps and caplets. In 1995, the Aum Shinrikyo cult used cyanide in train station restrooms with poor success.

Nomenclature

The term *cyanide* refers to the anion CN^-, or to its acidic form, hydrocyanic acid (HCN). Cyanogen (C_2N_2) is formed by the oxidation of cyanide ions; however, the term *cyanogen* has also come to refer to a substance that forms cyanide upon metabolism and produces the biological effects of free cyanide. Simple *cyanide* (HCN, NaCN) is a compound that dissociates to the cyanide anion (CN^-) and a cation (H, Na^+). A *nitrile* is an organic compound that contains cyanide. A cyanogen usually refers to a nitrile that liberates the cyanide anion during metabolism and produces the biological effects of the cyanide anion. Cyanogens may be simple (cyanogen chloride) or complex (sodium nitroprusside).

Cyanides are also called "blood agents," an antiquated term still used by many in the military. At the time of the introduction of cyanide in World War I, other chemical agents in use caused mainly local effects. In contrast, inhaled cyanide produces systemic effects and was thought to be carried in the blood, hence the term. The widespread distribution of absorbed nerve agents and vesicants via the blood invalidates this term as a specific designator for cyanide. Also, blood agent carries the connotation that the main site of action of cyanide is in the blood, whereas cyanide actually acts primarily outside the bloodstream.

Materials of interest as chemical agents are the cyanide *hydrogen cyanide* (HCN, AC) and the simple cyanogen *cyanogen chloride* (CK). Cyanogen bromide was used briefly in World War I but is of no present interest.

Sources Other Than Military

The cyanide ion is ubiquitous in nearly all living organisms that tolerate and even require the ion in low concentrations. The fruits and seeds (especially pits) of many plants of the Rosaceae family, such as cherries and peaches, as well as almonds and lima beans contain cyanogens capable of releasing free cyanide following enzymatic degradation. The edible portion (the roots) of the cassava plant (widely used as a food staple in many parts of the world) contains the cyanogenic glucoside linamarin. The combustion of any material containing carbon and nitrogen has the potential to form cyanide; some plastics (particularly acrylonitriles) predictably release clinically significant amounts when burned. Industrial concerns in the United States manufacture over 300,000 tons of hydrogen cyanide annually. Cyanides find widespread use in chemical syntheses, electroplating, mineral extraction, dyeing, printing, photography, agriculture, and in the manufacture of paper, textiles, and plastics.

Physiochemical Characteristics

The cyanides exist as liquids in munitions but rapidly vaporize upon detonation. The major threat is from vapor. The liquid's toxicity is approximately that of mustard. The low efficiency of cyanide on the battlefield has led to its disuse in combat operations.

Detection and Protection

The immediately dangerous to life and health (IDLH) concentration of AC is 50.0 parts per million (ppm); that for CK is 0.6 mg/m^3. The military detectors are capable of detecting AC and CK at the threshold limits given in Table 2-1.

Because the odor of cyanide may be faint or lost after accommodation, olfactory detection of the odor of bitter almonds is not a reliable indicator of cyanide exposure, even for those who possess the gene required to smell cyanide. The activated charcoal in the canister of the chemical protective mask adsorbs cyanide, and the mask affords full protection from this gas in an open field environment.

Table 2-1. Concentration Thresholds for Cyanide Detection

Detector	Concentration Threshold for AC (Hydrocyanic Acid)	Concentration Threshold for CK (Cyanogen Chloride)
JCAD	22.0 mg/m^3	20.0 mg/m^3
M256A1	7.0 mg/m^3	N/A

JCAD: Joint Chemical Agent Detector

Mechanism of Toxicity

Cyanide salts in solid form or in solution are readily absorbed from the gastrointestinal tract when ingested. Moreover, the lower the pH in the stomach, the more hydrogen cyanide is released as gas from ingested salts. Liquid cyanide and cyanide in solution can be absorbed even through intact skin, but this route of entry is usually not clinically significant. Parenteral absorption of liquid cyanide can also occur from wounds. Cyanide is readily absorbed through the eyes, but the most important route of entry in a battlefield or terrorist scenario is likely by inhalation. Following absorption, cyanide is quickly and widely distributed to all organs and tissues of the body. Ingestion leads to particularly high levels in the liver when compared with inhalation exposure, but both routes lead to high concentrations in plasma and erythrocytes and in the heart, lungs, and brain.

An example of the ability of cyanide to react with metals in the body is its reaction with the cobalt in hydroxycobalamin (vitamin B_{12a}) to form cyanocobalamin (vitamin B_{12}). The reactions of cyanide with metals are reversible and exhibit concentration-dependent equilibria, but the reactions of cyanide with sulfur-containing compounds are catalyzed by the enzyme rhodanese and are essentially one-way and irreversible. The rate-limiting factor in the rhodanese-mediated reactions is usually the availability of sulfur donors in the body. These reactions can be accelerated therapeutically by providing a sulfane such as sodium thiosulfate. The reaction products, thiocyanates and sulfites, are significantly less toxic than cyanide itself and are eliminated in the urine. Cyanide also reacts with carbonyl and sulfhydryl groups (directly or via 3-mercaptopyruvate sulfurtransferase and other enzymes). However, the two most important kinds of reactions to understand are the reactions with metals and the enzyme-catalyzed reactions with sulfur-containing compounds. Cyanide is eliminated unchanged from the body in breath, sweat, and urine. It is excreted as sodium thiocyanate in the urine and as iminothiocarboxylic acid from reaction with sulfhydryl groups at the cellular level. High concentrations of cyanide in the body also lead to measurable increases in urinary elimination of cyanocobalamin.

Toxicity

The LCt_{50} of AC by inhalation has been estimated to be half the LCt_{50} for CK. The median lethal dose (LD_{50}) for IV administration of hydrogen cyanide can be compared to a value of 1. Skin exposure is estimated to require a dose 100 times greater than IV for the same reaction. Oral exposure is estimated at 100 to 200 times greater than IV.

Cyanide is unique among military chemical agents because it is detoxified at a rate that is of practical importance, about 17 μg/kg•min. As a result, the LCt_{50} is greater for a long exposure (eg, 60 minutes) than for a short exposure (eg, 2 minutes).

Mechanism of Action

Cyanide has a high affinity for certain sulfur and certain metallic complexes, particularly those containing cobalt and the trivalent form of iron (Fe^{3+}). The cyanide ion can rapidly combine with iron in cytochrome a_3 (a component of the cytochrome aa_3 or cytochrome oxidase complex in mitochondria) to inhibit this enzyme, thus preventing intracellular oxygen utilization. The cell then utilizes anaerobic metabolism, creating excess lactic acid and a metabolic acidosis. Cyanide also has a high affinity for the ferric iron in methemoglobin, and one therapeutic stratagem induces the formation of methemoglobin to which cyanide preferentially binds.

The small quantity of cyanide always present in human tissues is metabolized at the approximate rate of 17 μg/kg•min, primarily by the hepatic enzyme rhodanese, which catalyzes the irreversible reaction of cyanide and a sulfane to produce thiocyanate, a relatively nontoxic compound excreted in the urine. (An elevated concentration of thiocyanate in either blood or urine is evidence of cyanide exposure.) The limiting factor under normal conditions is the availability of a sulfane as a substrate for rhodanese, and sulfur is administered therapeutically as sodium thiosulfate to accelerate this reaction. The lethal dose of cyanide is time dependent because of the ability of the body to detoxify small amounts of cyanide via the rhodanese-catalyzed reaction with sulfane. A given amount of cyanide absorbed slowly may cause no biological effects even though the same amount administered over a very short period of time may be lethal. In contrast, the LCt_{50} of each of the other chemical agents, which are not metabolized to the same extent as is cyanide, is relatively constant over time. A lethal amount causes death whether administered within minutes or over several hours.

Clinical Effects

The organs most susceptible to cyanide are those of the central nervous system (CNS) and the heart. Most clinical effects are of CNS origin and are nonspecific (Table 2-2). Approximately 15 seconds after inhalation of a high concentration of cyanide, there is a transient hyperpnea, followed within 15 to 30 seconds by the onset of convulsions. Respiratory activity stops 2 to 3 minutes later, and cardiac activity ceases several minutes later still, or approximately 6 to 8 minutes after exposure. The onset and progression of signs and symptoms after ingestion of cyanide or

Table 2-2. Effects From Cyanide (AC and CK) Vapor Exposure

Exposure	Signs and Symptoms	Course	Time
Moderate, from low concentration	Transient increase in rate and depth of breathing, dizziness, nausea, vomiting, headache.	These may progress to severe effects if exposure continues.	The time of onset of these effects depends on the concentration but is often within minutes after onset of exposure.
Severe, from high concentration	Transient increase in rate and depth of breathing, in 15 seconds. Convulsions, in 30 seconds. Cessation of respiration, in 2 to 4 minutes. Cessation of heartbeat, in 4 to 8 minutes.	Death if untreated.	Within seconds after onset of exposure.

after inhalation of a lower concentration of vapor are slower. The first effects may not occur until several minutes after exposure, and the time course of these effects depends on the amount absorbed and the rate of absorption.

The initial transient hyperpnea may be followed by feelings of anxiety or apprehension, agitation, vertigo, a feeling of weakness, nausea with or without vomiting, and muscular trembling. Later, consciousness is lost, respiration decreases in rate and depth, and convulsions, apnea, and cardiac dysrhythmias and standstill follow. Because this cascade of events is prolonged, diagnosis and successful treatment are possible.

The effects of cyanogen chloride, the parent complex of HCN, include those described for hydrogen cyanide. Cyanogen chloride is also similar to riot-control agents in causing irritation to the eyes, nose, and airways, as well as marked lacrimation, rhinorrhea, and bronchosecretions.

Physical findings are few and nonspecific. Two are said to be characteristic but in fact are not always observed. These are (1) severe respiratory distress in an acyanotic individual and "cherry-red" skin, and (2) the odor of bitter almonds. The natural complexion of the casualty may mask any cherry-red skin. When seen, cherry-red skin suggests either circulating carboxyhemoglobin from carbon monoxide poisoning or high venous oxygen content from failure of oxygen extraction by tissues poisoned by cyanide or hydrogen sulfide. However, cyanide victims may have normal-appearing skin or may be cyanotic, although cyanosis is not classically associated with cyanide poisoning. In addition, approximately 50% of the population is genetically unable to detect the odor of cyanide.

The casualty may be diaphoretic with normal sized or large pupils. A declining blood pressure and tachycardia follow an initial hypertension and compensatory bradycardia. Terminal hypotension is accompanied by bradyrhythmias before asystole.

Time Course of Effects

Effects begin 15 seconds following inhalation of a lethal Ct (concentration time); death ensues in about 6 to 8 minutes. The onset of effects following inhalation of lower Cts may be as early as minutes after the onset of exposure. After exposure is terminated by evacuation to fresh air or by masking, there is little danger of delayed onset of effects.

The time course for ingested cyanide is longer, with the victim initially complaining of stomach upset, due to the alkaline nature of potassium cyanide. This is followed after a period of approximately 7 minutes by hyperpnea, a feeling of anxiety in the patient, and within 15 minutes the patient feels weakness and experiences a loss of consciousness. Convulsions follow. Within 25 minutes apnea occurs, and soon the heart stops and death occurs. Typically, death occurs within 30 minutes after cyanide ingestion, depending on the dose ingested and the physiological make-up of the victim.

Differential Diagnosis

Inhalation exposure to either cyanide or a nerve agent may precipitate the sudden onset of loss of consciousness, followed by convulsions and apnea. The cyanide casualty has normal sized or dilated pupils, few secretions, and muscular twitching but no fasciculations. In contrast, the nerve agent casualty has miosis (until shortly before death), copious oral and nasal secretions, and muscular fasciculations. In addition, the nerve agent casualty may be cyanotic, whereas the cyanide casualty usually is not.

Laboratory Findings

There are several confirmatory laboratory tests for cyanide poisoning, listed below. However, due to rapid clinical deterioration, antidotal treatment must be provided immediately if signs and symptoms are clearly indicative of cyanide poisoning, rather than waiting for lab results.

- **An elevated blood cyanide concentration.** Mild effects may be apparent at concentrations of 0.5 to 1.0 $\mu g/mL$. Concentrations of 2.5 $\mu g/mL$ and higher are associated with coma, convulsions, and death and are used primarily for forensic confirmation.
- **Acidosis**. Metabolic acidosis with a high concentration of lactic acid (lactic acidosis) or metabolic acidosis with an

unusually high anion gap (if the means to measure lactic acid are not available) may be present. Because oxygen cannot be utilized, anaerobic metabolism with the production of lactic acid replaces aerobic metabolism. Lactic acidosis, however, may reflect other disease states and is not specific for cyanide poisoning. Test results are fairly rapid and valuable as an early confirmatory lab result.

- **Oxygen content of venous blood greater than normal**. This also is a result of poisoning of the cellular respiratory chain and the resulting failure of cells to extract oxygen from arterial blood. This finding is also not specific for cyanide poisoning. It is helpful in confirming a diagnosis and evaluating methemoglobin levels for later adjustments in the dose levels of methemoglobin-forming antidotes.

Medical Management

Management of cyanide poisoning begins with self-protection, then removal of the casualty to fresh air. Dermal decontamination is unnecessary if exposure has been to vapor only. With liquid exposure, wet clothing should be removed, and if liquid on the skin is a possibility, the underlying skin should be washed either with soap and water or with water alone. A casualty who has ingested cyanide does not require decontamination. In the case of ingestion, gavage and administer activated charcoal. All vomitous should be collected so that vapors from it do not sicken the staff.

Attention to the basics of intensive cardiorespiratory supportive care is critical and includes mechanical ventilation as needed, circulatory support with crystalloids and vasopressors, correction of metabolic acidosis with IV sodium bicarbonate, and seizure control with benzodiazepine administration. Administration of 100% oxygen has been found empirically to exert a beneficial effect and should be a part of general supportive care for the cyanide casualty.

Symptomatic patients, especially those with severe manifestations, may further benefit from specific antidotal therapy. This is provided in a two-step process. First, a methemoglobin-forming agent such as amyl nitrite (crushable ampoules for inhalation) or sodium nitrite (for IV use) is administered, because the ferric ion (Fe^{3+}) in methemoglobin has an even higher affinity for cyanide than does cytochrome a_3. The equilibrium of this reaction causes dissociation of bound cyanide from cytochrome a_3 and frees the enzyme to help produce adenosine triphosphate again. Hypotension, produced by nitrite administration, should be monitored. Further, there should be a prudent concern for overproduction of methemoglobin, which may compromise oxygen-carrying capacity. Thus, nitrite is relatively contraindicated in, for example, smoke-inhalation victims. In the standard cyanide antidote kit, the antidotes are already prepared in premeasured vials (amyl nitrite 1 ampule [0.2 mL] for 30–60 seconds; sodium nitrite 300 mg/10 mL of 3% solution); sodium thiosulfate 12.5 g [50 mL of 25% solution]). The initial adult dose, equivalent to one of the two sodium nitrite vials in the kit, is 10 mL. Pediatric nitrite dosing is dependent on body weight and hemoglobin concentration. The recommended pediatric dose, assuming a hemoglobin concentration of 12 g/dL, is 0.33 mL/kg of the standard 3% solution given slowly, IV, over 5 to 10 minutes.

The second step for treatment is the infusion of a sulfur donor, typically sodium thiosulfate, which is utilized as a substrate by rhodanese for its conversion of cyanide to thiocyanate. Sodium thiosulfate itself is efficacious, relatively benign, and also synergistic with oxygen administration. It may thus be used without nitrites empirically in situations such as smoke inhalation with high carboxyhemoglobin levels. The initial adult dose, equivalent to one of the two large bottles in the cyanide antidote kit, is 50 mL; the initial thiosulfate dose for pediatric patients is 1.65 mL/kg of the standard 25% solution, IV. Second treatments with each of the two antidotes may be given at up to half the original dose if needed. Directions are located on the inside of the kit lid.

Although the combination of sodium nitrite and sodium thiosulfate may save victims exposed to 10 to 20 lethal doses of cyanide and is effective even after breathing has stopped, many patients will recover even without specific antidotal treatment if vigorous general supportive care is provided. Lack of availability of antidotes is therefore not a reason to consider even apneic cyanide casualties expectant. It is also important to realize that administration of antidotes, especially if given too fast or in extremely large doses, is also associated with morbidity and even mortality. Antidotes should not be withheld in a patient with suspected cyanide poisoning, but infusion rates should be slow, and the drugs should be titrated to effect. Overdosage should be avoided.

Several alternative therapies and experimental antidotes are used in other NATO countries. Germany uses dimethylaminophenol, a rapid methemoglobin former developed for intramuscular and IV use. However, muscle necrosis at the site of injection may occur, and only the IV route of administration is recommended.

Certain cobalt compounds directly chelate cyanide to reduce its toxicity. Because cobalt compounds do not depend upon the formation of methemoglobin, they may exert their antidotal activity more quickly than do methemoglobin formers. Great Britain and France use cobalt edetate, but clear superiority to the methemoglobin formers has not been demonstrated, and cobalt toxicity is occasionally seen, particularly if the patient has only a mild exposure. The other cobalt compound sometimes used in France is hydroxocobalamin (vitamin B_{12a}), which forms a complex with cyanide on a molar basis. Clinical trials of this compound are underway in the United States. All of these compounds have been found to be most effective when combined with the administration of thiosulfate. Other ongoing research is examining whether slow methemoglobin formers can be used as pretreatment to induce clinically asymptomatic methemoglobinemia in troops at high risk for cyanide exposure.

Triage

Immediate casualties present within minutes of inhalation exposure with convulsions or recent onset of apnea. Circulation is intact. Immediate antidote administration is lifesaving.

Minimal casualties have inhaled less than a lethal amount and have mild effects. Antidotes may reduce symptoms but are not lifesaving.

Delayed casualties are recovering from mild effects or successful therapy. It may be hours before full recovery. Evacuation is not required.

Expectant casualties are apneic with circulatory failure or with a coexposure to other toxicants or trauma resulting in anoxic encephalopathy. Casualties may triage as expectant because of limited resources.

An inhalation exposure casualty who survives long enough to reach medical care will need little treatment. Respiratory support might be a basis for re-triage to a different category.

Return to Duty

Those with mild to moderate effects can usually return to duty within hours, and those successfully treated after severe effects can return within a day. Monitor for neurological damage caused by significant hypoxia.

Chapter 3

VESICANTS

Overview

Sulfur mustard (HD, H), the main focus of this chapter, has posed a military threat since its introduction on the battlefield in World War I. Unless otherwise noted, the term *mustard* refers here to sulfur mustard.

The nitrogen mustards (HN1, HN2, and HN3) were synthesized in the 1930s but were never produced in large amounts for warfare. Mechlorethamine (HN2, Mustargen [Recordati Rare Diseases, Lebanon, NJ]) became the prototypical cancer chemotherapeutic compound and remained the standard compound for this purpose for many years. Lewisite (L) was synthesized during the late stages of WWI but has probably not been used on a battlefield. The lewisite antidote, British anti-Lewisite (BAL; dimercaprol), finds medicinal use today as a heavy metal chelator. Although classified as a vesicant, phosgene oxime (CX) is a corrosive urticant that also has not seen battlefield use. Lewisite and phosgene oxime pose only minor potential military threats and will be discussed briefly at the end of this chapter.

MUSTARD

Summary

NATO Codes: H, HD

Signs and Symptoms: Asymptomatic latent period (hours). Erythema and blisters on the *skin;* irritation, conjunctivitis, corneal opacity, and damage in the *eyes;* mild upper respiratory signs to marked *airway* damage; also gastrointestinal effects and bone marrow stem cell suppression.

Field Detection: Joint Chemical Agent Detector (JCAD), M256A1 Chemical Agent Detector Kit, M18A2 Chemical Agent Detector Kit, Improved Chemical Agent Monitor (ICAM), M90 Chemical Warfare Agent Detector, M8 and M9 Chemical Agent Detector Paper, M21 Remote Sensing Chemical Agent Alarm (RSCAAL), M93 series Fox Reconnaissance System, M272 Chemical Agent Water Testing Kit, M22 Automatic Chemical Agent Detection Alarm (ACADA).

Decontamination: Reactive Skin Decontamination Lotion, 0.5% bleach solution, soap, and water in large amounts.

Management: Decontamination immediately after exposure is the only way to prevent damage. Supportive care of patients; there is no specific therapy.

Nomenclature

Sulfur mustard manufactured by the Levinstein process contains up to 30% impurities (mostly sulfur) and is known as H. Mustard made by a distillation procedure is almost pure and is known as HD (distilled mustard). An early term for the German agent was HS (probably derived from the World War I slang term *Hun Stoffe*).

Overview

Vesicant agents, specifically sulfur mustard (HD and H), constitute both a vapor and a liquid threat to all exposed skin and mucous membranes. Mustard's effects are delayed, appearing hours after exposure. The organs most commonly affected are the skin (with erythema and vesicles), eyes (with mild conjunctivitis to severe eye damage), and airways (with mild irritation of the upper respiratory tract to severe bronchiolar damage leading to necrosis and hemorrhage of the airway mucosa and musculature). Following exposure to large quantities of mustard, precursor cells of the bone marrow are damaged, leading to pancytopenia and increased susceptibility to infection. The gastrointestinal (GI) tract may be damaged, and there are sometimes central nervous system (CNS) signs. There is no specific antidote, and management is symptomatic therapy. Immediate decontamination is the only established way to reduce damage.

History and Military Relevance

Sulfur mustard was first synthesized in the early 1800s and was first used on the battlefield by Germany in July 1917. Despite its introduction late in World War I, mustard produced the most chemical casualties, although fewer than 5% of the casualties who reached medical treatment facilities died. Italy allegedly used mustard in the 1930s against Abyssinia. Egypt apparently employed mustard in the 1960s against Yemen, and Iraq used mustard in the 1980s against Iran and the Kurds. Most recently, in 2005, the Burmese military allegedly used a substance against the Karenni people of Burma causing many of the clinical symptoms seen in mustard victims. Accidental exposure from old ordinance also occurs frequently, with recent events in China in 2003 and Delaware in 2004. Mustard is still considered a major threat agent. The United States manufactured mustard during World War I and World War II. Most of its stockpile has been or is being destroyed.

Physiochemical Characteristics

Mustard is an oily liquid with a color ranging from light yellow to brown. Its odor is similar to garlic, onion, or mustard (hence its name), but because of accommodation of the sense of smell, odor should not be relied on for detection. Under temperate conditions, mustard evaporates slowly and is primarily a liquid hazard, but its vapor hazard increases with increasing temperature. At 100° F (37.7° C) or above, it is a definite vapor hazard. Mustard freezes at 57°F (13.9°C), and since a solid is difficult to disperse, mustard is often mixed with substances with a lower freezing point such as lewisite (the mixture is called HL), so that the mixture will remain liquid at lower temperatures. The mixture HT refers to mustard that has been thickened with small quantities of newer thickening agents to make it even more persistent.

Detection and Protection

The immediately dangerous to life and health (IDLH) concentration of sulfur mustard (H) is 0.003 mg/m^3. Liquid mustard turns M8 paper a ketchup red, and M9 paper will turn pink, red, reddish-brown, or purple when exposed to liquid nerve agents or vesicants, but does not specifically identify either the class of agent or the specific agent. Because the odor of sulfur mustard may be faint or lost after accommodation, olfactory detection of the odor of mustard, garlic, onions, or horseradish is not a reliable indicator of mustard exposure. The detectors in the Table 3-1 have the capacity to detect sulfur mustard at the threshold limits given.

The activated charcoal in the canister of the US Army chemical protective mask adsorbs mustard, as does the charcoal in the chemical protective overgarment. The butyl rubber in the chemical protective gloves and boots is impermeable to mustard. Proper wear of the chemical protective mask and the chemical protective ensemble affords full protection against sulfur mustard.

Table 3-1. Concentration Thresholds for Sulfur Mustard Detection*

Detector	Concentration Threshold
JCAD	2.0 mg/min^3
M256A1	3.0 mg/min^3
M272 (in water)	2.0 mg/min^3
M18A2	0.5 mg/min^3
M21	150 mg/min^3
M90	0.2 mg/min^3
M93A1 Fox	0.01–1.00 μg/L
ICAM	0.1 mg/min^3

*Values change with updated versions; please refer to the manufacturer for the most up to date thresholds.

JCAD: Joint Chemical Agent Detector
ICAM: Improved Chemical Agent Monitor

Mechanism of Toxicity

Mustard vapor and liquid readily penetrate thin layers of most fabrics (but not the chemical protective ensemble) to reach underlying skin. Although mustard dissolves relatively slowly in aqueous solutions such as sweat, the lipophilicity of mustard guarantees effective absorption through even intact skin. Penetration is rapid (1 to 4 $\mu g/cm^2/min$) and is enhanced by moisture, heat, and thin skin. This explains the otherwise baffling observation that World War I mustard burns involved the scrotum in 42% of cases, but the presumably more readily exposed hands in only 4% of cases. Ocular and respiratory routes of entry are also important, as is parenteral absorption in casualties with conventional wounds. Ingestion (enteral absorption) was an important route of entry in the sailors who jumped into mustard floating on the sea from an exploding ship that carried the agent, the SS *John Harvey*, docked at Bari Harbor, Italy, during World War II.

Approximately 10% of the amount of mustard that begins penetrating the skin will bind to the skin as "fixed" (reacted) mustard; the remaining 90% of the dose reaches the circulation and is systemically distributed as "free" (unreacted and hydrolyzed) mustard. Mustard is distributed to almost all the organs and tissues, including kidneys, liver, intestines, and lungs, although, because of dilutional effects and reactions of mustard in the bloodstream, clinical effects from systemic distribution are seen only at high doses. After intravenous (IV) administration, mustard disappears from the blood within seconds to minutes. Because of the rapid fixation of mustard to tissue, the fluid inside the blisters that eventually develop at the sites of skin contact contains no free mustard and does not pose a contamination hazard to healthcare providers.

Mustard participates in a variety of biotransformative (metabolic) reactions in the body. Some of these reactions are catalyzed by enzymes, but most absorbed mustard reacts directly by forming covalent bonds (via alkylation) with DNA, RNA, proteins, components of cell membranes, and other macromolecules in the body. Mustard is eliminated primarily in the urine as a byproduct of alkylation.

Toxicity

The median lethal concentration (LCt_{50}) of sulfur mustard dispersed as a vapor in an unprotected group is approximately six times more lethal than in a group with respiratory protection. This demonstrates not only the importance of respiratory protection, but also the fact that sufficient concentrations of vapor and sufficient exposure times render mustard vapor lethal, even in masked individuals. The median lethal dose (LD_{50}) of liquid mustard on the skin is about the amount of a teaspoon or a single condiment yellow mustard packet. Although a teaspoon of a liquid applied evenly to the surface of the skin may cover approximately 20% to 25% of the total body surface area (BSA), the correlation between BSA involvement and deaths from mustard in the field is poor. One plausible reason for this discrepancy is that using BSA figures alone ignores the inhalational component of mustard exposure.

Another conceivable explanation is that measurement solely of affected BSA neglects factors such as the thickness of coverage, subsequent spread, contact time, and continued exposure. A 10 μg droplet of sulfur mustard can produce a small vesicle on exposed skin.

Toxicodynamics (Mechanism of Action)

Absorbed mustard must first dissolve in an aqueous solution such as sweat or extracellular fluid. Although mustard molecules dissolve slowly in such solutions, once dissolved they rapidly (within seconds to a minute or two) rearrange to form extremely reactive cyclic ethylene sulfonium ions that immediately bind to intracellular and extracellular enzymes, proteins, and other cellular components. Mustard has many biological actions, but the exact mechanism by which it produces tissue injury is not certain. According to one prominent hypothesis, biological damage from mustard results from DNA alkylation and crosslinking in rapidly dividing cells, such as basal keratinocytes, mucosal epithelium, and bone marrow precursor cells. This leads to cellular death and inflammatory reaction, and in the skin, protease digestion of anchoring filaments at the epidermal-dermal junction and the formation of blisters. Mustard also possesses mild cholinergic activity, which may be responsible for effects such as early GI symptoms and miosis.

It should be reemphasized that mustard reacts with tissue within minutes of entering the body and that blood, tissue, and blister fluid do not contain free mustard, nor do they represent a contamination risk for medical personnel.

Clinical Effects

Topical effects of mustard occur in the eye, airway, and skin (Table 3-2). Systemically absorbed mustard may produce effects in the bone marrow, GI tract, and CNS. Direct injury to the GI tract may also occur following ingestion of the compound. Combined data from US forces in World War I and Iranians in the Iran-Iraq conflict suggest equal incidence of eye, airway, and skin involvement (between 80% and 90% for each). However,

Table 3-2. Effects of Mustard Vapor

Organ	Severity	Effects	Onset
Eye	Mild	Tearing, itchy, burning, gritty feeling	4–12 hours
	Moderate	Above, plus reddening, swelling of lids, moderate pain	3–6 hours
	Severe	Marked swelling of lids, possible cornea damage, severe pain	1–2 hours
Airways	Mild	Runny nose, sneezing, nosebleed, hoarseness, hacking cough	12–24 hours
	Severe	Above, plus severe productive cough, shortness of breath	2–4 hours
Skin	Mild to severe	Erythema (redness), blisters	2–24 hours

incidences of eye and lung damage were higher in Iranian casualties than in World War I casualties, probably because of the agent's increased evaporation in the hot climate.

Skin

Erythema is the mildest and earliest form of skin injury after exposure to mustard. It resembles sunburn and is associated with pruritus or burning, stinging pain. Erythema begins to appear in 2 to 48 hours after vapor exposure with time of onset dependent on concentration-time product (Ct), ambient temperature and humidity, and skin site exposed. The skin sites most sensitive are the warm, moist locations with thinner skin such as the perineum, external genitalia, axillae, antecubital fossae, and neck.

Within the erythematous areas, small vesicles can develop that may later coalesce to form bullae. The typical bulla, or blister, is large, dome-shaped, thin-walled, translucent, yellowish, and surrounded by erythema. The blister fluid is clear, at first thin and straw-colored but later yellowish and tending to coagulate. The fluid does not contain mustard and is not a vesicant.

At extremely high doses such as those from liquid exposure, lesions may develop a central zone of coagulation necrosis with blister formation at the periphery. These lesions take longer to heal and are more prone to secondary infection than the uncomplicated lesions seen at lower exposure levels.

Pulmonary

The primary airway lesion from mustard is necrosis of the mucosa, with later damage to the airway musculature if the amount of agent is large. The damage begins in the upper airways and descends to the lower airways in a dose-dependent manner. Usually the terminal airways and alveoli are affected only as a terminal event. Pulmonary edema is not usually present unless the damage is very severe, and then it is usually hemorrhagic.

The earliest effects from mustard, perhaps the only effects from a low Ct, involve the nose, sinuses, and pharynx. There may be irritation or burning of the nares, epistaxis, sinus pain or irritation, and irritation or soreness of the pharynx. As the Ct increases, other effects occur, such as laryngitis with voice changes and a nonproductive cough, and damage to the trachea and upper bronchi leading to a cough productive of sputum. Lower airway involvement causes dyspnea and an increasingly severe cough with increased quantities of sputum. Terminally, there may be necrosis of the smaller airways with hemorrhagic edema into surrounding alveoli (although this hemorrhagic pulmonary edema is rare).

Necrosis of the airway mucosa with resulting inflammation can cause pseudomembrane formation. Pseudomembranes may occur from the most proximal parts of the airways to the most distal portions. These membranes may cause local airway restriction at the sites of formation, and detachment may lead to obstruction of lower airways.

The cause of death in mustard poisoning is commonly respiratory failure. Mechanical obstruction by pseudomembranes and agent-induced laryngospasm are important causes of death in the first 24 hours after exposure. Deaths occurring from the third to the sixth day after exposure result from secondary bacterial pneumonia caused by bacterial invasion of denuded respiratory mucosa and necrotic debris. Agent-induced bone marrow suppression is a contributory factor in later, septic deaths from pneumonia.

Eyes

The eyes are the organs most sensitive to mustard vapor injury. The latent period is shorter for eye injury than for skin injury and is also Ct dependent. After low-dose vapor exposure, irritation evidenced by reddening of the eyes may be the only effect. As the dose increases, the spectrum of injury includes progressively more severe conjunctivitis, photophobia, blepharospasm, pain, and corneal damage.

Blisters do not normally form in the eyes. Instead, swelling and loosening of corneal epithelial cells lead to corneal edema and clouding with leukocytes (which affects vision). Corneal vascularization with secondary edema may last for weeks. Scarring between the iris and lens may follow severe effects; this scarring may restrict pupillary movements and may predispose victims to glaucoma.

The most severe damage is caused by liquid mustard from airborne droplets or by self-contamination. After extensive eye exposure, severe corneal damage with possible perforation of the cornea and loss of the eye can occur. Eye loss also results from panophthalmitis if appropriate therapy is not instituted. Miosis noted after mustard exposure in both humans and experimental animals is probably from the cholinomimetic activity of mustard.

During World War I, mild conjunctivitis accounted for 75% of eye injuries, with recovery in 1 to 2 weeks. Moderate conjunctivitis with minimal corneal involvement, blepharospasm, edema of the lids and conjunctivae, and orange-peel roughening of the cornea accounted for 15% of the cases, with recovery in 4 to 6 weeks. Severe corneal involvement accounted for 10% of the cases. Those with permanent corneal damage accounted for less than 1% of cases. About 0.1% of these severe casualties would meet the criteria for legal blindness today.

Gastrointestinal Tract

The mucosa of the GI tract is very susceptible to mustard damage, from either systemic absorption or ingestion of the agent. However, reports of severe GI effects from mustard poisoning are relatively infrequent. Mustard exposure, even exposure to a small amount, will often cause nausea, with or without vomiting, lasting 24 hours or less. However, the nausea and vomiting appear to result not from the agent's effects on the GI tract, but rather from a stress reaction, a nonspecific reaction to the odor, or cholinergic stimulation by mustard. Further GI symptoms are usually minimal unless the exposure was severe (even then, GI signs are not common) or resulted from ingestion of contaminated food or drink. Diarrhea has been reported; constipation is equally common. Diarrhea (rarely bloody) and vomiting beginning days after a high-dose exposure imply a poor prognosis.

Central Nervous System

The CNS effects of mustard remain poorly defined. Animal research has demonstrated that mustards (particularly the nitrogen mustards) are convulsants, and several human case reports describe victims exposed to very large amounts who had neurological effects within several hours after exposure, just prior to death. Reports from World War I, and again from Iran, described people exposed to small amounts of mustard who appeared sluggish, apathetic, and lethargic. These reports suggest that minor psychological problems could linger for a year or longer.

Time Course of Effects

Mustard binds irreversibly to tissue and causes tissue damage within several minutes of contact without causing any concomitant clinical effects such as burning or erythema. To prevent injury, *decontamination must be carried out immediately after contact*. If decontamination is not carried out immediately after exposure, there is no way to prevent injury. Because of the lack of immediate effects, the contaminated person is often unaware of the exposure and does not decontaminate. Later decontamination may prevent further damage, absorption, or spread of the agent.

After a high-dose exposure, signs and symptoms may appear

as early as 2 hours after contact. Following a low-dose vapor exposure, the latent or asymptomatic period may extend to 48 hours. There are several reports of individuals exposed to very large amounts who died within hours; this type of occurrence is extremely rare. The typical onset time is between 4 and 8 hours. The concentration of the mustard vapor, time of exposure, ambient weather, and body site exposed are factors in onset time.

Differential Diagnosis

Of the three vesicant agents, mustard is the only one that does not cause immediate pain. The casualty is asymptomatic until the lesion becomes apparent hours later. Lewisite and phosgene oxime, in contrast, cause immediate pain or irritation to the eye, skin, or respiratory tract, which is sufficient stimulus to decontaminate immediately or to mask.

Isolated small blisters or a small group of blisters suggest possible exposure to mustard as well as to plants such as poison ivy or poison oak, drugs, or other substances. The physical characteristics of the lesion are not distinctive; therefore, the history of exposure is invaluable. Although the blisters of mustard and lewisite are slightly different (there is less erythema around the lewisite blister), this distinction is of little value in individual cases.

Laboratory Findings

Leukocytosis occurs during the first day, and the magnitude of increase in leukocytes during subsequent days correlates roughly with the amount of tissue injury, primarily to skin or pulmonary tissue. If systemic absorption is large, leukocytes in the peripheral blood will decrease beginning on day 3 to day 5; this decrease indicates damage to precursor cells in the blood-forming organs. The decrease may be precipitate, for example, a decrease of 5,000 to 10,000 cells per day. If the marrow damage is severe, erythrocytes and thrombocytes may decrease later, but the casualty usually recovers or dies before this is apparent. A leukocyte count of 500 or fewer is a sign of an unfavorable prognosis.

Signs of a chemical pneumonitis may appear within the first 2 to 3 days after inhalation exposure. Leukocytosis, fever, and sputum production suggest a bacterial process, but within this time period sputum cultures are usually negative for pathogens. Organisms commonly invade the damaged airway tissue at days 3 to 5. A change in the fever pattern, an increase in leukocytosis, and a change in the character of the sputum in this time period suggest a bacterial process. Sputum Gram stain and culture should be done for identification of the specific organism. Damaged skin should be cultured routinely, particularly if there is an increase in the exudate or in the inflammatory reaction.

Although GI bleeding is unusual, declining hematocrit values should prompt serial analyses of stool for occult blood. Thiodiglycol, a urinary metabolite of sulfur mustard, can be measured in a deployed Army medical laboratory. There is no clinical laboratory test for mustard in blood or tissue, nor is one expected since mustard is biotransformed and bound to tissues within minutes after absorption. However, ways to measure blood and tissue adducts produced in the body after reaction with sulfur mustard are being studied.

Medical Management

The management of a patient exposed to mustard may be simple, as in providing symptomatic care for a sunburn-like erythema, or extremely complex, as in providing total management for a severely ill patient with burns, immunosuppression, and multisystem involvement. Suggested therapeutic measures for each organ system are provided below. Guidelines for general patient care are not intended to take the place of sound clinical judgment, especially in the management of complicated cases.

Skin

Erythema should be treated with calamine or another soothing lotion or cream (eg, 0.25% camphor and menthol) to reduce burning and itching. Small blisters (under 1–2 cm) should be left intact, but because larger ones will eventually break (the blister fluid does not contain mustard), they should be carefully unroofed, or the fluid can be aspirated. Denuded areas should be irrigated three to four times daily with saline, another sterile solution, or soapy water and then liberally covered with a topical antibiotic such as silver sulfadiazine or mafenide acetate to a thickness of 1 to 2 mm. If an antibiotic cream is not available, sterile petrolatum may be useful. Modified Dakin solution (sodium hypochlorite) was used in World War I and in Iranian casualties for irrigation and as an antiseptic. Multiple or large areas of vesication suggest the need for hospitalization and whirlpool bath irrigation.

Systemic analgesics should be used liberally, particularly before manipulation of the patient or irrigation of the burn areas. Systemic antipruritics such as trimeprazine should be tried if needed. Monitoring of fluids and electrolytes is important in any sick patient, but it must be recognized that fluid loss is not of the magnitude seen with thermal burns. Clinicians accustomed to treating patients with thermal burns must resist the temptation to overhydrate a mustard casualty with a similar amount of burned body surface.

Eyes

Conjunctival irritation from a low Ct will respond to any of a number of available ophthalmic solutions after the eyes are thoroughly irrigated. Regular application of homatropine (or other anticholinergic drug) ophthalmic ointment will reduce or prevent future synechiae formation. A topical antibiotic applied several times a day will reduce the incidence and severity of infection. Vaseline or a similar substance should be applied to the edges of the lids regularly to keep them from sticking together. This prevents adhesions and later scarring during healing and also permits drainage of any underlying infection or pus. Topical analgesics may be useful initially if blepharospasm is too severe to permit an adequate examination, but topical analgesics should otherwise be avoided, and systemic analgesics should be given for eye pain. Topical steroids are not of proven value, but their use during the first day or two might reduce inflammation. Further use should be left to an ophthalmologist. Sunglasses may reduce discomfort from photophobia. The patient should be constantly reassured that complete healing and restoration of vision will be the outcome.

Pulmonary

Upper airway symptoms (sore throat, nonproductive cough, and hoarseness) may respond to steam inhalation and cough suppressants. Although a productive cough and dyspnea accompanied by fever and leukocytosis occurring 12 to 24 hours after exposure may suggest a bacterial process, clinicians must resist the urge to use antibiotics to treat these symptoms, which result from sterile bronchitis or pneumonitis. Infection often occurs on about the third day. Its presence is signaled by an increased fever, an increase in the pulmonary infiltrate by x-ray, and an increase in sputum production and change in sputum character to purulent. Appropriate antibiotic therapy should await confirmation of the clinical impression by positive sputum studies (Gram stain and culture).

Intubation should be performed early, before laryngeal spasm or edema makes it difficult or impossible. Intubation permits better ventilation and facilitates suction of the necrotic and inflammatory debris. Oxygen may be needed, and early use of positive end-expiratory pressure or continuous positive airway pressure may be of benefit. If there is a suggestion of pseudomembrane formation, bronchoscopy should be performed to permit suctioning of the necrotic debris by direct vision.

Bronchodilators may be of benefit for bronchospasm. If they fail, steroids may be tried. There is little evidence that the routine use of steroids is beneficial. The need for continuous use of assisted or controlled ventilation suggests a poor prognosis.

Death often occurs between the 5th and 10th day after exposure because of pulmonary insufficiency and infection complicated by a compromised immune response from agent-induced bone marrow damage.

Gastrointestinal

Atropine (0.4–0.6 mg, intramuscular or IV), another anticholinergic drug, or an antiemetic should control the early nausea and vomiting. Prolonged vomiting or voluminous diarrhea beginning days after exposure suggests direct involvement of the GI tract by severe systemic poisoning, a poor prognostic sign.

Bone Marrow

Alteration of gut flora by nonabsorbable antibiotics should be considered to reduce the possibility of sepsis from enteric organisms. Cellular replacement (bone marrow transplants or transfusions) may be successful, because intact mustard does not persist beyond the few minutes following absorption and would not damage the new cells.

General

A patient severely ill from mustard poisoning requires the general supportive care provided for any severely ill patient, as well as the specific care given to a burn patient. Liberal use of systemic analgesics and antipruritics, as needed, maintenance of fluid and electrolyte balance, and other supportive measures are necessary. Parenteral nutrition and supplements, including vitamins, may also be helpful.

In studies, sulfur donors such as sodium thiosulfate decreased systemic effects and elevated the LD_{50} when given before exposure or within 20 minutes after exposure in experimental tests. Activated charcoal given orally to casualties was of no value. Hemodialysis was not only ineffective, but actually harmful in several casualties. The rapid biotransformation of the mustard molecule suggests that none of these measures would be beneficial hours or days after exposure.

Triage

Most mustard casualties will be triaged as *delayed*. Those with skin lesions covering a small percentage to half of the BSA require further medical care but do not need immediate lifesaving assistance. (In contrast, patients with thermal burns covering 20% to 70% of BSA are considered immediate because of their fluid requirements.) Those with mild to moderate pulmonary effects will also eventually require further care but are not in the immediate category for triage. Eye injuries from other causes require immediate care, but by the time the mustard eye lesion develops, there is no possibility of reducing the injury. These casualties are also in the delayed category.

Patients with skin lesions covering a small percentage of BSA (under 5%) when the lesions are not in vital areas (eg, a burn on the face might prevent mask donning) are triaged as *minimal.* Clinical judgment should dictate whether these patients should be evacuated for care or whether they can return to duty. The tactical situation will also be a factor in the decision. Patients with minor eye injuries including irritation and reddening can be treated and returned to duty. Those with slight upper respiratory complaints such as a hacking cough and irritated throat that developed 12 hours or longer after exposure might be given symptomatic therapy and returned to duty.

The only mustard casualties who might be triaged as *immediate* are those with moderately severe to severe pulmonary signs and symptoms. Two factors should temper this decision. First, casualties who develop severe pulmonary effects within 4 to 6 hours of exposure will probably not survive despite maximal medical care, and it might be better to expend limited medical resources elsewhere. Second, if evacuation to a higher role of care is required, some casualties may survive the lengthy trip, but their lesions may progress to an irreversible stage during the delay.

A mustard casualty who has severe pulmonary effects that developed within 4 to 6 hours of exposure should be triaged as *expectant.* A casualty who has over 50% BSA burns from mustard liquid might also be categorized as expectant, but this decision depends on available medical resources at the far rear roles of medical care. (The LD_{50} for liquid mustard is about a teaspoon of liquid. This amount will cover about 25% BSA, so an individual with a 50% BSA burn could possibly have two LD_{50} lesions on his or her skin. This person might be saved, but at great expenditure of medical resources.)

Long-Term Effects

Repeated symptomatic exposures to mustard over a period of years (such as manufacturing workers might experience) seem to be well established as a causal factor in an increased incidence of upper-airway cancer. However, the association between a single exposure to mustard and airway cancer is not well established. A single, severe exposure to mustard may have contributed to other airway problems, such as chronic bronchitis, in World War I casualties. A new complication seen in Iranian casualties from the Iran-Iraq War in the 1980s was late-onset tracheobronchial stenosis, which presumably would have been seen in World War I casualties had antibiotic therapy been available to save the lives of those who died from secondary bacterial pneumonia.

Several eye diseases, such as chronic conjunctivitis and delayed keratitis, may follow a single severe exposure of the eye to mustard. Skin scarring and pigment changes may follow a severe skin lesion from mustard, and cancer sometimes develops in scarred skin.

Mustard is classed as a mutagen and carcinogen, based on laboratory studies. However, there are no data to implicate mustard as a reproductive toxin in humans, and there is no evidence that mustard is a causative factor in nonairway, non-skin cancer in humans.

Supplemental Considerations for Treatment and Disposition

In addition to the treatment modalities cited above, ongoing research on the management of mustard injuries and observation of sulfur mustard accidents that occurred in the United States and abroad has resulted in the information summarized below. The only major information on human mustard casualties is from World War I and the Iran-Iraq conflict in the 1980s because human mustard injury research is unethical.

Eye

Research at the US Army Medical Research Institute of Chemical Defense (USAMRICD) has shown remarkable results using steroids and antibiotic eye combinations. Eyes that would have been nearly destroyed appeared almost normal when these combinations were applied early and frequently. In the study, the treatments were given both by injection and topically in the form of solutions and ointments. The results were so remarkable that commercially available ophthalmologic steroid and antibiotic solutions or ointments were recommended for inclusion in the field medical sets. The recommended application is as soon as possible in connection with even the mildest mustard eye injury. The frequency of use is every 1 to 2 hours until the full extent of the developing mustard injury becomes known. The treatment should then be modified accordingly, with consultation and examination by an ophthalmologist as soon as possible. This initial treatment should be applied only in the absence of a penetrating injury to the eye or in the case of obvious, secondary bacterial infection. Narcotic analgesia may be used if eye pain is severe.

Exposure to sulfur mustard can lead to a chronic eye inflammation with associated pain, erosions, and even frank ulceration. This keratitis has been seen to develop as early as 8 months and as late as 20 years after initial exposure. It does not seem to be associated with severity of exposure, although a higher incidence with more severe exposures may be expected. Mustard-induced chronic keratitis was either infrequent or undetected in the years following World War I.

Pulmonary

No specific antidotes for mustard injury to the lung exist; however, standard supportive care should be employed for all pulmonary injuries. Mustard injuries to the trachea and bronchi have a high rate of secondary bacterial infection starting as early as 3 days and developing as late as 2 to 3 weeks after exposure. Late development is especially frequent with doses leading to significant bone marrow depression. Prophylactic administration of antibiotics is contraindicated and will lead to the selection of resistant bacterial infections. Vigilant lookout for the early signs and symptoms of infection, and Gram stain and cultures to aid selection of the most appropriate antibiotic, are key.

The sloughing of necrotic bronchial mucosa, as pseudomembranes or as amorphous debris, can be severe enough to cause mechanical blockage and suffocation. Soldiers in World War I died from these blockages. Treatment is rigorous percussion, postural drainage, and provision of humidified air with supplemental oxygen. At times, fiberoptic bronchoscopy may be needed to remove the blockage.

A complication not reported from World War I, but seen in casualties from the Iran-Iraq War in the 1980s, is severe tracheobronchial stenosis. Bronchospasm with asthma-like symptoms can be a frequent complication of the mustard lung injury. The medicines used for the bronchospasm are the same as with asthma: β-adrenergic dilators, steroids, and theophylline-type drugs. Steroidal antiinflammatory agents have never been scientifically shown to be beneficial in cases of mustard lung injury. However, if β-adrenergic bronchodilators do not provide complete relief, many clinicians would be quick to add steroids to aid in ending the bronchospasm. Again, caution is warranted because of the likelihood of secondary bacterial infection in cases of exposure to sulfur mustard.

With significant irritation to the larynx, acute closure caused by laryngospasm is possible and may result in death if a patent airway is not maintained. Pulmonary edema is not a normal feature of mustard lung injury except in cases of very large exposures, when hemorrhagic pulmonary edema may be seen. Mounting circumstantial evidence suggests the possibility of chronic bronchial disease developing after significant pulmonary exposure.

Mustard is a proven carcinogen, but no cases of cancer have been documented with acute exposures. However, some factory workers chronically exposed to low doses of sulfur mustard in World War I developed cancers of the respiratory tract (nasopharynx, larynx, and lung). A small amount of laboratory data in rats and mice points to reproductive abnormalities. Anecdotal stories about reproductive abnormalities are now coming out of Iran and Iraq, but these will take years to substantiate with good epidemiological studies. The possibility of a causal link between mustard exposure and late onset or chronic health effects should always be investigated in patients with a documented or suspected history of exposure.

Skin

Vesication may take several days to complete. Mustard blister fluid does *not* contain active sulfur mustard. Once a patient has been adequately decontaminated, medical personnel do not have to fear contamination. Mustard casualties with skin injury may require narcotics for analgesia.

Mustard skin burns are generally more superficial than thermal burns, but the services of an intensive care unit or surgical burn unit may be a necessity. Judicious IV fluid and electrolyte therapy are required with significant mustard skin burns, but fluid requirements are less than with corresponding thermal burns. Fluids and electrolytes should be closely monitored because fluids may be lost to edematous areas, with resultant dehydration. Medical personnel are cautioned not to over-hydrate the patient because hypervolemia and pulmonary edema can be iatrogenically induced in mustard casualties. The exact fluid replacement requirements for cutaneous mustard injuries should be based on patient status and considered on a case-by-case basis.

Multiple techniques exist for caring for mustard skin burns / blisters / wounds: (*a*) leaving the blisters intact; (*b*) removing or debriding the roof of large blisters; (*c*) leaving the blister roof intact and aspiring the fluid with a sterile needle; or (*d*) removing the blister roof and temporarily covering it with artificial or pig skin. A universal measure is the use of a topical antibiotic cream or ointment whether the blister is intact or not. The topical antibiotic depends on individual experience and preference, starting with traditional surgical preparations and working down to whatever is available. A moist wound-healing environment should be maintained during the reepithelialization process for optimal outcome. Initially, the attachment of the neoepidermis to the underlying dermis may be weak, and protective dressings may be needed to avoid or minimize damage as a result of friction with clothing or bedding.

The tremendous inflammation caused by sulfur mustard in human skin can easily be confused with bacterial cellulitis; however, mustard skin wounds can easily develop a secondary bacterial cellulitis, requiring the use of appropriate systemic antibiotics. Infection surveillance and specialty consultation may be necessary.

It has long been recognized that mustard skin wounds are slow to heal, taking sometimes twice the time that would be expected with a conventional wound or a thermal burn. The hypothesis explaining these observations is that abnormal compounds of DNA (DNA adducts) are produced, delaying the healing time. Also, the skin histologically very often looks more like scar tissue than normal skin. Recent studies in the United States (USAMRICD) and England (Porton Down) have shown that appropriate debridement of the deeper mustard burns leads to more normal healing times and return to regular skin architecture. Good results were obtained with both laser debridement and traditional mechanical techniques. Accurate depth assessment is important, because it dictates how aggressive treatment must be to minimize or prevent cosmetic and functional deficits (eg, deep injuries will need to be excised and grafted). Microcutaneous blood flow is a good prognostic indicator and should be monitored using laser Doppler perfusion imaging or indocyanine green fluorescence imaging.

Bone Marrow

Sulfur mustard, like nitrogen mustard and certain chemotherapeutic compounds, is an alkylating agent. Systemic absorption of sulfur mustard above what would be 25% of a lethal dose can lead to significant bone marrow depression. This is why the systemic effects of sulfur mustard have been described as radiomimetic. The earliest indicator that a patient may have received a significant systemic exposure is nausea and vomiting persisting longer than the first hour or 2 after exposure. Nausea and vomiting 24 hours later is definitely a warning sign. The next most sensitive indicator is a fall in the lymphocyte count; this lymphopenia may occur as early as the first 24 hours. The polymorphonuclear cell count may actually rise in the first 24 hours. Other cellular components of blood may show a significant decline as early as 3 days after exposure, and patients can be in profound marrow suppression by 1 to 3 weeks following exposure. The usual life-threatening complication is sepsis and septic pneumonia. Transfusions, isolation techniques, hormonal stimulation of the marrow, and appropriate antibiotics may all be utilized.

Studies in nonhuman primates conducted by the US Navy using nitrogen mustard and by the US Army with sulfur mustard showed an improved bone marrow recovery time using granulocyte colony stimulating factor (GCSF). GCSF is a commercially available product for use in standard cases of marrow suppression.

Gastrointestinal

Severe hemorrhagic diarrhea may be caused either by direct ingestion of sulfur mustard or by systemic absorption following exposure by other routes. High doses of sulfur mustard can induce necrosis and sloughing of the GI mucosa. The most important aspect of treatment is IV fluids and electrolytes. Anticholinergics to control bowel spasm and possibly narcotic analgesia are indicated if acute surgical abdomen is not a complication. Hemorrhage may be severe enough to require transfusion.

Central Nervous System

In the first few hours after exposure to sulfur mustard, patients may experience mood swings ranging from depression to euphoria. The mechanism for these mood changes is not understood. Supportive care is indicated. A few individuals in World War I who received massive exposures to sulfur mustard experienced seizures and died rapidly. This phenomenon has also been observed in animals.

Return to Duty

Casualties with minor skin, eye, or pulmonary injuries might be returned to duty as soon as they are given symptomatic therapy at a medical facility. The range of return-to-duty times for those with more severe but treatable injuries is from a week to a year or longer. Those with eye injuries should recover in 1 to 3 weeks, except for the low percentage of casualties with severe injuries or complications. Casualties with mild to moderate pulmonary injuries should return to duty in a week to a month. Healing of mild skin lesions will enable the casualty to return within several weeks, but patients with large skin lesions will require hospitalization for many months. Because of the slow healing of sulfur mustard injuries, casualties with significant injury to the eyes, respiratory tract, skin, GI tract, or CNS will not return to duty for weeks to months.

Eye

Only individuals with the mildest eye irritations to sulfur mustard will be able to return to duty. The mildest form of conjunctivitis causes a functional blindness caused by pain, photophobia, and spasm of the eyelid muscles; this conjunctivitis takes an average of 2 weeks to resolve. As the severity of the injury increases, so does the time for healing. A moderate conjunctivitis may require 2 full months before return to duty is possible. In rare instances, blindness may result from severe exposures.

Lung

Only individuals experiencing an irritation without significant tissue injury will be able to return to duty. Determining whether patients have received only an irritation or the mildest of injuries will require 3 to 7 days of observation. Anyone with documented mustard lung injury producing a bronchial pneumonia or pseudomembrane formation will not be able to return to duty for several months. Those with severe cases may never return to duty.

Skin

Only casualties with lesions on a small percentage of BSA (less than 5%) in noncritical areas will be able to return to duty following treatment with topical antibiotic, dressings, and oral analgesics. Burns to the hands, feet, face, axillae, and groin are all potentially disabling. Return to duty will require weeks to months in all but the mildest of injuries.

Burns by liquid on the skin and in the eye cause the most severe injury. It is possible in some instances to receive a nearly total body burn from mustard vapor with effects no more severe than those from second-degree sunburn. A vapor burn of this milder level of severity takes 48 hours or more to develop. However, a vapor burn developing in only a few hours could be as severe as a liquid burn. Severity of a mustard burn is dependent upon the total absorbed dose of vapor and liquid.

Guidelines for Medical Evacuation

A casualty who requires hospital care for longer than 2 weeks, specialty care not available in theater, or intensive care or burn center-level treatment should be medically evacuated as soon as feasible to a Role 3 or 4 facility.

Physical Examination, Laboratory, and Procedures at Role 5

These recommendations pertain *only* to patients requiring Role 5 care. There should be a full, appropriate internal medicine, dermatology, ophthalmology, or burn surgical examination on admission. Serial evaluations should focus on any abnormalities until they are resolved with time and appropriate treatment. Patients with injury involving specific organ systems (eyes, respiratory tract, GI tract, blood, or CNS) should receive consultative care by the appropriate specialists.

Return to duty should be delayed until after full recovery. Temporary duties during convalescence should be appropriate to the patient's condition until full return to duty or medical retirement. After full recovery, the patient should have follow-up evaluations every 6 months with appropriate studies for specific injuries. If problems are found, appropriate care should be given, with return visits as frequently as necessary. After two 6-month follow-up visits showing no problems, the patient should be reevaluated annually for 5 years. Any associated medical problems will extend the period of close follow-up until complete resolution or maximal medical improvement.

In the absence of related medical problems at 5 years, the patient may be discharged to an as-needed follow-up status. However, patients with a mustard eye injury should undergo ophthalmology evaluations every 5 years (or more frequently as needed) for life, and patients with mustard pulmonary injury (larynx, nasopharynx, trachea, and lung) should undergo a pulmonary evaluation as clinically indicated, and at least every 5 years, for life. Also, patients who have recovered from pancytopenia caused by sulfur mustard should be refered to a hematologist as indicated and at a mnimum every 5 years, for life.

LEWISITE

Summary

NATO Code: L

Signs and Symptoms: Lewisite causes immediate pain or irritation of skin and mucous membranes. Erythema and blisters on the skin and eye and airway damage similar to conditions seen after mustard exposures develop later.

Field Detection: Joint Chemical Agent Detector (JCAD), M256A1 Chemical Agent Detector Kit, M18A2 Chemical Agent Detector Kit, Improved Chemical Agent Monitor (ICAM), M90 Chemical Warfare Agent Detector, M8 and M9 Chemical Agent Detector Paper, M21 Remote Sensing Chemical Agents Alarm (RSCAAL), M93 series Fox Reconnaissance System, M272 Chemical Agent Water Testing Kit, M22 Automatic Chemical Agent Detection Alarm (ACADA).

Decontamination: Reactive Skin Decontamination Lotion, soap and water, 0.5% bleach solution.

Management: Immediate decontamination; symptomatic management of lesions is the same as for mustard lesions; a specific antidote (BAL) will decrease systemic effects.

Overview

Lewisite (L) is a vesicant that damages the eyes, skin, and airways by direct contact. After absorption, it causes an increase in capillary permeability that produces hypovolemia, shock, and organ damage. Exposure to lewisite causes immediate pain or irritation, although lesions require hours to become full-blown. Management of a lewisite casualty is similar to management of a mustard casualty, although a specific antidote, BAL, will alleviate some pathophysiological effects.

History and Military Relevance

Dr. Wilford Lee Lewis first synthesized lewisite in 1918, too late for its use in World War I. It has not been used in warfare, although some countries may stockpile it. Lewisite is sometimes mixed with mustard to achieve a lower freezing point of the mixture for ground dispersal and aerial spraying.

Physiochemical Characteristics

Lewisite is an oily, colorless liquid with the odor of geraniums. It is more volatile than mustard.

Detection and Protection

The IDLH concentration of lewisite is 0.003 mg/m^3. The M8A1 Automatic Chemical Agent Detector Alarm cannot detect lewisite. However, liquid lewisite turns M8 paper red, and M9 paper turns pink, red, reddish-brown, or purple when exposed to liquid nerve agents or vesicants, but does not specifically identify either the class of agent or the specific agent. The detectors in Table 3-3 can detect lewisite at the threshold limits given.

Because the odor of lewisite may be faint or lost after accommodation, olfactory detection of the odor of geraniums is not a reliable indicator of exposure. The activated charcoal in the canister of the chemical protective mask adsorbs lewisite, as does the charcoal in the chemical protective overgarment. Lewisite attacks the butyl rubber in the chemical protective gloves and boots, which are expected to protect against field concentrations of lewisite until they can be exchanged for fresh gloves and boots. Proper wear of the chemical protective mask and ensemble affords full protection against lewisite.

Mechanism of Toxicity

Lewisite is readily absorbed through the skin, eyes, and respiratory tract, as well as by ingestion and via wounds. It is systemically distributed to almost all organs and tissues of the

Table 3-3. Concentration Thresholds for Lewisite Detection*

Detector	Concentration Threshold
JCAD	2.0 mg/min^3
M256A1	14.0 mg/min^3
M272 (in water)	2.0 mg/min^3
M18A2	10.0 mg/min^3
M21	150.0 mg/min^3
M90	0.2 mg/min^3
M93 series Fox	10–100 μg/L
ICAM	2.0 mg/min^3

*Values change with updated versions; please refer to the manufacturer for the most up to date thresholds.
JCAD: Joint Chemical Agent Detector
ICAM: Improved Chemical Agent Monitor

body, where it participates in a variety of chemical reactions. It is eventually eliminated primarily as reaction products in the urine.

Toxicity

Lewisite causes nasal irritation at a Ct of about 8 mg•min/m^3, and its odor is noted at a Ct of about 20 mg•min/m^3. Lewisite causes vesication and death from inhalation at the same Ct as mustard. Liquid lewisite causes vesication at about 14 μg, and the LD_{50} of liquid lewisite applied to the skin is about half that of mustard.

Mechanism of Action

Although lewisite contains trivalent arsenic and combines with thiol groups in many enzymes, its exact mechanism of action is unknown.

Clinical Effects

Unlike mustard, lewisite vapor or liquid causes *immediate* pain or irritation. A person with a droplet of lewisite on the skin will feel burning and immediately try to remove the substance. The vapor is so irritating that those affected will seek to mask or leave the contaminated area if possible. These immediate steps may lessen severity of lewisite lesions as compared to mustard, because exposure to mustard is often undetected and decontamination is often delayed. There are almost no data on humans exposed to lewisite. The following information is based on laboratory investigations.

Skin

Within about 5 minutes after contact, liquid lewisite will produce a grayish area of dead epithelium. Erythema and blister formation follow more rapidly than in a similar lesion from mustard, although the full lesion does not develop for 12 to 18 hours. The lesion develops more tissue necrosis and tissue sloughing than does a mustard lesion.

Eye

Lewisite causes pain and blepharospasm on contact. Edema of the conjunctiva and lids follows, and the eyes may be swollen shut within an hour. Iritis and corneal damage may follow if the dose is high. Liquid lewisite causes severe eye damage within minutes of contact.

Pulmonary

The extreme irritancy of lewisite to the central airway compartment causes the person to mask or exit the area. Lewisite may cause the same airway signs and symptoms as mustard. The airway mucosa is the primary target, and damage progresses down the airways in a dose-dependent manner. Pseudomembrane formation is prominent. Pulmonary edema, which occurs rarely and usually only to a minimal degree after mustard exposure, may complicate exposure to lewisite.

Other Symptoms

Available data suggest that lewisite causes an increase in permeability of systemic capillaries with resulting intravascular fluid loss, hypovolemia, shock, and organ congestion. This may lead to hepatic or renal necrosis with more prominent GI effects (including vomiting and diarrhea) than after mustard. Physical findings are similar to those caused by mustard. Tissue damage at the site of the skin lesion may be more severe.

Time Course of Effects

Pain and irritation from either liquid or vapor lewisite are immediate. Early tissue destruction is more obvious than after mustard, but the lesion is not full-blown for 12 hours or longer.

Differential Diagnosis

Although differences have been reported between the skin lesions from mustard and lewisite (less surrounding erythema and more tissue destruction characterize lewisite blisters), these are of little diagnostic assistance. The history of immediate pain on contact is absent after mustard exposure and present after lewisite or phosgene oxime exposures. Other substances also cause erythema and blisters, and often the history of exposure is the most helpful tool in diagnosis.

Laboratory Findings

There is no specific diagnostic test for lewisite. Leukocytosis, fever, and other signs of tissue destruction will occur.

Medical Management

Early decontamination is the only method of preventing or lessening lewisite damage. This self-aid must be accomplished within minutes after exposure. Medical treatment follows the guidelines for mustard casualty management. Lewisite does not cause damage to hematopoietic organs as mustard does; however, fluid loss from the capillaries necessitates careful attention to fluid balance.

BAL is an antidote for lewisite and is used as a chelating agent for heavy metals. There is evidence that BAL in oil, given intramuscularly, will reduce the systemic effects of lewisite. However, BAL itself has some toxicity, and the user should read the package insert carefully. BAL skin and ophthalmic ointment decreases the severity of skin and eye lesions when applied immediately after early decontamination; however, neither is currently manufactured.

Triage

Triage using the guidelines for mustard.

Return to Duty

Casualties with minor skin lesions who receive symptomatic therapy can be returned to duty quickly. Because lewisite generally causes more tissue damage than mustard, casualties with eye and larger skin lesions should be triaged as *delayed* and evacuated. Pulmonary injury casualities may be triaged as immediate, delayed, or expectant depending on the severity of the injury and time of onset.

PHOSGENE OXIME

Summary

NATO Code: CX

Signs and Symptoms: Immediate burning and irritation followed by wheal-like skin lesions and eye and airway damage.

Field Detection: Joint Chemical Agent Detector (JCAD), M256A1 Chemical Agent Detector Kit, M18A2 Chemical Agent Detector Kit, M90 Chemical Warfare Agent Detector, M93 series Fox Reconnaissance System.

Decontamination: Reactive Skin Decontamination Lotion, soap and water, 0.5% bleach solution.

Management: Immediate decontamination, symptomatic management of lesions.

Overview

Phosgene oxime (CX) is an urticant or nettle agent that causes a corrosive type of skin and tissue lesion. It is not a true vesicant because it does not cause blisters. The vapor is extremely irritating, and both the vapor and liquid cause almost immediate tissue damage upon contact. There is very scanty information available on CX.

Military Significance

There is no current assessment of the potential of CX as a military threat agent.

Physiochemical Characteristics

Phosgene oxime is a solid at temperatures below 95° F (35° C), but the vapor pressure of the solid is high enough to produce symptoms. Traces of many metals cause it to decompose; however, it corrodes most metals.

Detection and Protection

The IDLH concentration of CX has not been defined. M8 and M9 paper should not be depended upon to detect this agent. The M256A1 detector ticket reacts to the presence of CX, but the detection threshold is not known with certainty. The detectors in Table 3-4 are capable of detecting CX at the threshold limits given. Because the odor of phosgene may be faint or lost after accommodation, olfactory detection of a pepperish or pungent odor is not a reliable indicator of the presence of CX. The activated charcoal in the canister of the chemical protective mask adsorbs CX, as does the charcoal in the chemical protective overgarment. Phosgene oxime may attack the butyl rubber in the chemical protective gloves and boots, which nevertheless are expected to protect against field concentrations of CX until they can be exchanged for fresh gloves and boots. Proper wear of the chemical protective mask and chemical protective ensemble affords full protection against CX.

Table 3-4. Concentration Thresholds for Phosgene Oxime Detection*

Detector	Concentration Threshold
M18A2	0.5 mg/min^3
M90	0.15 mg/min^3
M93A1 Fox	10–100 $\mu g/L$

*Values change with updated versions; please refer to the manufacturer for the most up to date thresholds.

Mechanism of Toxicity

The toxicokinetics of CX are not known in detail. Penetration of exposed surfaces is rapid, and systemic distribution to most organs and tissues, including the GI tract, is probably important.

Toxicity

The estimated LCt_{50} by inhalation is approximately the same as mustard. The LD_{50} for skin exposure has been estimated as approximately three to four times as much as mustard, or about 3 to 4 teaspoons.

Toxicodynamics (Mechanism of Action)

The mechanism by which CX causes biological effects is unknown.

Clinical Effects

Skin

Phosgene oxime liquid or vapor causes pain on contact, which is followed in turn by blanching with an erythematous ring in 30 seconds, a wheal in 30 minutes, and necrosis later. Extreme pain may persist for days.

Eye

Phosgene oxime is extremely painful to the eyes. The damage is probably similar to that caused by lewisite.

Pulmonary

Phosgene oxime is very irritating to the upper airways. This agent causes pulmonary edema after inhalation and after skin contact.

Other

Some animal data suggest that CX may cause hemorrhagic inflammatory changes in the GI tract.

Time Course of Effects

Phosgene oxime causes immediate pain and irritation to all exposed skin and mucous membranes. The time course of damage to other tissue probably parallels that of damage to the skin.

Differential Diagnosis

Other causes of urticaria and skin necrosis must be considered. Common urticants do not cause the extreme pain of CX exposure.

Laboratory Findings

There are no distinctive laboratory findings.

Medical Management

Management is supportive. The skin lesion should be managed in the same way that a necrotic ulcerated lesion from another cause would be managed.

Triage

Because of continuing pain, most casualties should be placed in the *delayed* category and evacuated.

Return to Duty

The decision to return a CX casualty to duty should be based on healing of the lesions and resolution of discomfort.

Chapter 4

NERVE AGENTS

Summary

NATO Codes: GA, GB, GD, GF, VX

Signs and Symptoms:
Vapor, small dose: miosis, rhinorrhea, mild difficulty breathing.
Vapor, large dose: sudden loss of consciousness, convulsions, apnea, flaccid paralysis, copious secretions, miosis.
Liquid on skin, small to moderate dose: localized sweating, nausea, vomiting, feeling of weakness.
Liquid on skin, large dose: sudden loss of consciousness, convulsions, apnea, flaccid paralysis, copious secretions.

Field Detection: Joint Chemical Agent Detector (JCAD), M256A1 Chemical Agent Detector Kit, M18A2 Chemical Agent Detector Kit, M8 Chemical Agent Detector Paper, M9 Chemical Agent Detector Paper, Improved Chemical Agent Monitor (ICAM), M93 series Fox Reconnaissance System, M21 Remote Sensing Chemical Agent Alarm (RSCAAL), M90 Chemical Warfare Agent Detector, M22 Automatic Chemical Agent Detection Alarm (ACADA).

Decontamination: Reactive Skin Decontamination Lotion, soap and water, 0.5% hypochlorate solution.

Management: Administer three Antidote Treatment Nerve Agent Autoinjectors (ATNAAs) and one Convulsive Antidote, Nerve Agent (CANA) to severe casualties; support airway for respiratory distress.

Overview

Nerve agents are the most toxic of the known chemical agents. They are hazards in both liquid and vapor states and can cause death within minutes after exposure. Nerve agents inhibit acetylcholinesterase in tissue, and their effects are caused by the resulting excess acetylcholine.

History and Military Relevance

Nerve agents were developed in pre-World War II Germany. Germany had stockpiles of nerve agent munitions during World War II but did not use them for reasons that remain unclear. In the closing days of the war, the United States and its allies discovered these stockpiles, developed the agents, and manufactured nerve agent munitions. The US chemical agent stockpile, which is in the process of being destroyed, contains the nerve agents sarin (GB) and VX.

Nerve agents are considered major military threat agents. The only known battlefield use of nerve agents was in the Iraq-Iran conflict. Syria's chemical agent stockpile is a major concern. Intelligence analysts indicate that many countries have the technology to manufacture nerve agent munitions.

Physical Characteristics

Nerve agents are liquids under temperate conditions. When dispersed, the more volatile nerve agents constitute both a vapor and a liquid hazard. Others are less volatile and represent primarily a liquid hazard. The G-agents (agents discovered by Germany) are more volatile than VX. GB is the most volatile, but it evaporates less readily than water. GF is the least volatile of the G-agents.

Nerve agents can be dispersed from many types of ground- and air-based munitions as both a vapor and liquid. These include but are not limited to mortars, missiles, rockets, grenades, landmines, and spray tanks.

Detection and Protection

The immediately dangerous to life and health concentrations of nerve agents are 0.0001 mg/m^3 for tabun (GA), 0.0001 mg/m^3 for GB, 0.0003 mg/m^3 for soman (GD), 0.0001 mg/m^3 for GF, and 0.0001 mg/m^3 for VX. Liquid G-agents turn M8 paper a gold yellow, and VX turns M8 paper dark green or olive green. M9 paper will turn pink, red, reddish brown, or purple when exposed to liquid nerve agents or vesicants but does not specifically identify either the class of agent or the specific agent. See Table 4-1 for detection threshold limits by detector and agent.

Because the odor of nerve agents may be faint or lost after accommodation, olfactory detection of the odor of fruit or fish is not a reliable indicator of exposure. The activated charcoal in the canister of the chemical protective mask adsorbs nerve agents present as vapor or gas, as does the charcoal in the chemical protective overgarment. The butyl rubber in the chemical protective gloves and boots is impermeable to nerve agents. Proper wear of the protective mask and the chemical protective ensemble affords full protection against nerve agents.

Table 4-1. Threshold Limits for Nerve Agent Detection

Detector	GA (Tabun)	GB (Sarin)	GD (Soman)	GF	VX
JCAD	1.0 mg/m^3	1.0 mg/m^3	1.0 mg/m^3	0.1 mg/m^3	0.041mg/m^3
M256A series	Unknown	0.05 mg/m^3	Unknown	Unknown	0.02 mg/m^3
M90	< 0.1 mg/m^3	< 0.1 mg/m^3	< 0.1 mg/m^3	< 0.1 mg/m^3	< 0.1 mg/m^3
ICAM	0.03 mg/m^3	0.03 mg/m^3	0.03 mg/m^3	0.03 mg/m^3	0.01 mg/m^3
M22	0.001 PPM	0.002 PPM	0.002 PPM	Unknown	0.0009 PPM

ICAM: Improved Chemical Agent Monitor; JCAD: Joint Chemical Agent Detector; PPM: parts per million

Mechanism of Toxicity

Nerve agents are organophosphorus cholinesterase inhibitors. They inhibit the butyrylcholinesterase in plasma, acetylcholinesterase in red blood cells, and acetylcholinesterase at cholinergic receptor sites in tissue. The three enzymes are not the same; even the two acetylcholinesterases have slightly different properties, although both have a high affinity for acetylcholine. Measuring blood enzymes provides an estimate of the tissue enzyme activity. After acute exposure to a nerve agent, the erythrocyte enzyme activity most closely reflects the activity of the tissue enzyme, but during recovery the plasma enzyme activity more closely parallels tissue enzyme activity.

After a nerve agent inhibits the tissue enzyme, the enzyme cannot hydrolyze acetylcholine, the neurotransmitter, at cholinergic receptor sites. Acetylcholine accumulates and continues to stimulate the affected organ. Organs with cholinergic receptor sites include the smooth muscles, skeletal muscles, central nervous system (CNS), and most exocrine glands. In addition, cranial efferents and ganglionic afferents are cholinergic nerves. The clinical effects from nerve agent exposure are caused by excess acetylcholine.

Muscarine will stimulate some of the cholinergic sites, and these are known as muscarinic sites. Organs with these sites include the smooth muscles and glands. Nicotine will stimulate other cholinergic sites, known as nicotinic sites, which are those in skeletal muscle and ganglia. The CNS contains both types of receptors, but the pharmacology in the CNS is more complex and less well understood. Atropine and similar compounds block the effects of excess acetylcholine more effectively at muscarinic sites than at nicotinic sites.

Some commonly used organophosphate and carbamate pesticides and some common therapeutic drugs (the carbamates pyridostigmine and physostigmine) also inhibit acetylcholinesterase and can be considered nerve agents. However, while the organophosphate pesticides cause the same biological effects as traditional nerve agents discussed here, there are some important differences in the duration of biological activity and response to therapy.

The attachment of the agent to the enzyme is permanent (unless removed by therapy). Erythrocyte enzyme activity returns at the rate of erythrocyte turnover, about 1% per day. Tissue and plasma enzyme activities return with synthesis of new enzymes. The rate of return of the tissue and plasma enzymes is not the same, nor is the rate the same for all tissue enzymes. However, the agent can be removed from the enzyme and the enzyme "reactivated" by several types of compounds, the most useful of which are the oximes. If the agent-enzyme complex has not "aged" (a biochemical process by which the agent-enzyme complex becomes refractory to oxime reactivation of the enzyme), oximes are useful therapeutically. For most nerve agents, the aging time is longer than the time before acute casualties will be seen by a healthcare provider. However, the aging time of the GD-enzyme complex is about 2 minutes, and the usefulness of oximes in GD poisoning is greatly decreased after this period.

Clinical Effects

The initial effects of exposure to a nerve agent depend on the dose and route of exposure. The initial effects from a sublethal amount of agent by vapor exposure are different from the initial effects from a similar amount of liquid agent on the skin. The estimated amounts to cause certain effects in humans are shown

Table 4-2. Comparative Nerve Agent Vapor Toxicity*

Agent	LCt_{50}	ICt_{50}	MCt_{50}
GA	400	300	2–3
GB	100	75	3
GD	70	Unknown	< 1
GF	Unknown	Unknown	< 1
VX	50	35	0.04

*For this table, one concentration of VX = 50, and one concentration of GB = 100, meaning it would take 2 times more GB to have the same median lethal dose as one concentration of VX.
LCt_{50}: median lethal concentration/time
ICt_{50}: median incapacitation concentration/time
MCt_{50}: median first noticeable effect (of miosis) concentration/time

Table 4-3. Comparative Median Lethal Dose Values on Skin*

Agent	Amount
GA	100
GB	170
GD	5
GF	3
VX	1

*Refer to FM 3-11.9, *Potential Military Chemical/Biological Agents and Compounds*, for specific LD_{50} information. For this table, one dose of VX = 1, and 170 doses of GB = 170, meaning it would take 170 times more GB to have the same median lethal dose as one dose of VX.

in Tables 4-2 (vapor) and 4-3 (liquid on skin). The large amounts of GA and GB required to produce effects after skin application reflect the volatility of these agents; they evaporate rather than penetrate the skin. However, if these agents are occluded and prevented from evaporating, they penetrate the skin very well. GB, the agent studied most thoroughly in humans, causes miosis, rhinorrhea, and a feeling of tightness in the throat or chest at a concentration of 3 to 5 mg•min/m^3.

Exposure to a small amount of nerve agent vapor causes effects in the eyes, nose, and airways. These effects are from local contact of the vapor with the organ and do not indicate systemic absorption of the agent. In this circumstance, the erythrocyte cholinesterase may be normal or depressed. A small amount of liquid agent on the skin causes systemic effects initially in the gastrointestinal (GI) tract. Lethal amounts of vapor or liquid cause a rapid cascade of events culminating within a minute or two with loss of consciousness and convulsive activity, followed by apnea and muscular flaccidity within several more minutes.

Eye

Miosis is a characteristic sign of exposure to nerve agent vapor. It occurs as a result of direct contact of vapor with the eye. Liquid agent on the skin will not cause miosis if the amount of liquid is small. A moderate amount of liquid may or may not cause miosis. A lethal or near-lethal amount of agent usually causes miosis.

A droplet of liquid in or near the eye will also cause miosis. Miosis will begin within seconds or minutes after the onset of exposure to agent vapor, but it may not be complete for many minutes if the vapor concentration is low. Miosis is bilateral in an unprotected individual, but occasionally may be unilateral in a masked person with a leak in one eyepiece.

Miosis is often accompanied by complaints of pain, dim vision, blurred vision, nausea, occasional vomiting, and the presence of conjunctival injection. The pain may be sharp or dull, in or around the globe, but most often there is a dull ache in the frontal part of the head. Dim vision is due in part to the constricted pupil, and cholinergic mechanisms in the visual pathways also contribute. The complaint of blurred vision is less easily explained, because objective testing usually indicates an improvement in visual acuity because of the "pin-hole" effect caused by the miosis (the "pin-hole" effect results from blocking peripheral light waves, which are most distorted by refractive error, from entering the eye, reducing the blur by allowing only the most central light rays to reach the retina and providing clearer vision). Conjunctival injection may be mild or severe, and occasionally subconjunctival hemorrhage is present. Nausea (and sometimes vomiting) is part of a generalized complaint of not feeling well. Topical homatropine or atropine in the eye can relieve miosis, pain, dim vision, and nausea.

Nose

Rhinorrhea may be the first indication of nerve agent vapor exposure. Its severity is dose dependent.

Airway

Nerve agent vapor causes bronchoconstriction and increased secretions of the glands in the airways in a dose-related manner. The exposed person may feel a slight tightness in the chest after a small amount of agent and may be in severe distress after a large amount of agent. Cessation of respiration occurs within minutes after the onset of effects from exposure to a large amount of nerve agent. This apnea is probably mediated through the CNS, although peripheral factors (skeletal muscle weakness, eg, in the intercostal muscles, and bronchoconstriction) may contribute.

Gastrointestinal Tract

After absorbtion, nerve agents cause an increase in the GI tract's motility and an increase in secretions by the glands in the GI tract's walls. Nausea and vomiting are early signs of liquid exposure on the skin. Diarrhea may occur with exposure to large amounts of agent.

Glands

Nerve agent vapor causes increases in secretions from the glands it contacts, such as the lacrimal, nasal, salivary, and bronchial glands. Localized sweating around the site of liquid agent on the skin is common, and generalized sweating after a large liquid or vapor exposure is common. Increased secretions of the glands of the GI tract occur after systemic absorption of the agent by either route.

Skeletal Muscle

The first effect of nerve agents on skeletal muscle is stimulation, producing muscular fasciculations and twitching. After a large amount of agent, muscle fatigue and weakness is rapidly followed by muscular flaccidity. Fasciculations are sometimes seen early at the site of a droplet of liquid agent on the skin, and generalized fasciculations are common after a large exposure. These may remain long after most of the other acute signs decrease.

Central Nervous System

The acute CNS signs of exposure to a large amount of nerve agent are loss of consciousness, seizure activity, and apnea. These begin within a minute after exposure to vapor and may be preceded by an asymptomatic period of 1 to 30 minutes after contact of liquid with the skin.

After exposure to smaller amounts of nerve agent, CNS effects vary and are nonspecific. They may include forgetfulness, an inability to concentrate fully, insomnia, bad dreams, irritability, impaired judgment, and depression. These may occur in the absence of physical signs or other symptoms of exposure. After a severe exposure, these symptoms occur upon recovery from the acute severe effects. In either case, they may persist for as long as 4 to 6 weeks. CNS effects do not include frank confusion and misperceptions (ie, hallucinations).

Cardiovascular

The heart rate may be decreased because of stimulation by the vagus nerve, but it is often increased because of other factors such as fright, hypoxia, and the influence of adrenergic stimulation secondary to ganglionic stimulation. Thus, the heart rate may be high, low, or in the normal range. Bradyarrhythmias such as first-, second-, or third-degree heart block may occur. The blood pressure may be elevated from adrenergic factors, but it is generally normal until the terminal decline.

Physical Findings

Physical findings depend on the amount and route of exposure. After exposure to small to moderate amounts of vapor, there are usually miosis and conjunctival injection, rhinorrhea, and pulmonary signs, although the latter may be absent even in the face of mild to moderate pulmonary complaints. In addition to these signs, an exposure to a high Ct (concentration-time product) may precipitate copious secretions from the nose and mouth, generalized muscular fasciculations, twitching or seizure activity, loss of consciousness, and apnea. Cyanosis, hypotension, and bradycardia may be present just before death.

Exposure to a small droplet of liquid on the skin may produce few physical findings. Sweating, blanching, and occasional fasciculations at the site may be present soon after exposure, but may no longer be present at the onset of GI effects. After a large exposure, the signs are the same as after vapor exposure. Miosis is a useful sign of exposure to vapor but does not occur after a liquid exposure unless the amount of exposure is large or the exposure is in or close to the eye.

Time Course of Effects

Effects from nerve agent vapor (Table 4-4) begin within seconds to several minutes after exposure. Loss of consciousness and onset of seizure activity have occurred within a minute of exposure to a high Ct. After exposure to a very low Ct, miosis and other effects may not begin for several minutes, and miosis may not be complete for 15 to 30 minutes after removal from the vapor. There is no latent period or delay in onset from vapor exposure. Effects may continue to progress for a period of time, but maximal effects usually occur within minutes after exposure stops.

A large amount of liquid on the skin causes effects (Table 4-5) within minutes. Commonly there is an asymptomatic period of 1 to 30 minutes, and then the sudden onset of an overwhelming cascade of events, including loss of consciousness, seizure activity, apnea, and muscular flaccidity. After small amounts of liquid agent on the skin, the onset of effects has been delayed for as long as 18 hours after contact. These effects are initially

Table 4-4. Nerve Agent Effects: Vapor Exposure

Mild • Eyes: miosis, dim vision, headache • Nose: rhinorrhea • Mouth: salivation • Lungs: dyspnea (tightness in the chest) • Time of onset: seconds to minutes after exposure	**Immediate Treatment** • *Self-aid:* one ATNAA • *Buddy-aid:* stand by
Severe All of the above, plus • Severe breathing difficulty or cessation of respiration • Generalized muscular twitching, weakness, or paralysis • Convulsions • Loss of consciousness • Loss of bladder and bowel control • Time of onset: seconds to minutes after exposure	**Immediate Treatment** • *Self-aid:* none; soldier will be unable to help self • *Buddy-aid:* three ATNAAs and diazepam immediately

ATNAA: antidote treatment nerve agent autoinjector

Table 4-5. Nerve Agent Effects: Liquid on Skin

Mild to Moderate	Immediate Treatment
• Muscle twitching at site of exposure • Sweating at site of exposure • Nausea, vomiting • Feeling of weakness • Time of onset: 10 minutes to 18 hours after exposure	• *Self-aid*: one to two ATNAAs, depending on severity of symptoms • *Buddy-aid:* stand by
Severe	**Immediate Treatment**
All of the above, plus • Severe breathing difficulty or cessation of breathing • Generalized muscular twitching, weakness, or paralysis • Convulsions • Loss of consciousness • Loss of bladder and bowel control • Time of onset: minutes to an hour after exposure	• *Self-aid*: none; soldier will be unable to help self • *Buddy-aid*: three ATNAAs and diazepam immediately

ATNAA: antidote treatment nerve agent autoinjector

gastrointestinal and are usually not life-threatening. Generally, the longer the interval, the less severe the effects.

Differential Diagnosis

The effects caused by a mild vapor exposure, namely, rhinorrhea and tightness in the chest, may easily be confused with an upper respiratory malady or allergy. Miosis, if present, will help to distinguish exposure from these diseases, but the eyes must be examined in very dim light to detect it. Similarly, GI symptoms from another illness may be confused with those from nerve agent effects, and in this instance there will be no useful physical signs. History of possible exposure will be helpful, and laboratory evidence (decreased red blood cellcholinesterase activity), if available, will be useful to make the distinction. Diagnosis is easier in the severely intoxicated patient. The combination of miosis, copious secretions, and generalized muscular fasciculations in a gasping, cyanotic, and convulsing patient is characteristic.

Laboratory Findings

Nerve agents inhibit the cholinesterase activity of the blood components, and estimation of this activity is useful in detecting exposure. The erythrocyte enzyme activity is more sensitive to acute nerve agent exposure than is plasma enzyme activity. The amount of inhibition of enzyme activity does not correlate well with the severity of local effects from mild to moderate vapor exposure. The enzyme activity with localized exposure may be from 0% to 100% of the individual's normal activity, causing miosis, rhinorrhea, and/or airway symptoms. Normal or nearly normal erythrocyte acetylcholinesterase activity may be present, with moderate local effects in the exposed tissue. At the other extreme, the enzyme may be inhibited by 60% to 70% when miosis or rhinorrhea is the only sign of exposure. Severe systemic effects generally indicate inhibition of the erythrocyte acetylcholinesterase by 70% to 80% or greater. Other laboratory findings will relate to complications. For example, acidosis may occur after prolonged hypoxia.

Medical Management

Managing a casualty with nerve agent intoxication consists of decontamination, ventilation, administration of antidotes, and supportive therapy. The condition of the patient dictates the need for each of these measures and the order in which they are done. Decontamination is described elsewhere in this manual. Skin decontamination is not necessary after exposure to vapor alone, but clothing should be removed because it may contain trapped vapor.

The need for ventilation will be obvious, and the means of ventilation will depend on available equipment. Bronchoconstriction and secretions increase airway resistance (to 50 to 70 cm of water), making initial ventilation difficult. The resistance decreases after atropine administration, after which ventilation is easier. However, the copious secretions may be thickened by atropine, impeding ventilatory efforts and requiring frequent suctioning. In reported cases of severe nerve agent exposure, ventilation has been required from 0.5 to 3 hours.

Three drugs (atropine, pralidoxime chloride, and diazepam) are used to treat nerve agent exposure, and another (pyridostigmine bromide) is used as pretreatment for potential nerve agent exposure. Atropine is a cholinergic-blocking or anticholinergic compound. It is extremely effective in blocking the effects of excess acetylcholine at peripheral muscarinic sites. When small amounts (2 mg) are given to healthy individuals without nerve agent intoxication, atropine causes mydriasis, a decrease in secretions (including a decrease in sweating), mild sedation, a decrease in GI motility, and tachycardia. In the military, atropine is packaged in autoinjectors, each containing 2 mg. The atropine dose in three ATNAAs may cause adverse effects on military performance in an unexposed person, and amounts of 10 mg or more may cause delirium. Potentially, the most hazardous effect of inadvertent use of atropine (2 mg, intramuscular) in a young person not exposed to a cholinesterase-inhibiting compound in a warm or hot atmosphere is inhibition of sweating, which may lead to heat injury.

Pralidoxime chloride (2-PAMCl) is an oxime. Oximes attach to the nerve agent inhibiting the cholinesterase and break the agent-enzyme bond to restore the normal activity of the enzyme. Clinically, this is noticeable in organs with nicotinic receptors. Abnormal activity in skeletal muscle decreases and normal strength returns. The effects of an oxime are not apparent in organs with muscarinic receptors; oximes do not cause a decrease in secretions, for example. They also are less useful after aging occurs, but with the exception of GD-intoxicated individuals, casualties would be treated before significant aging occurs. In addition to the atropine autoinjectors, the ATNAAs contain an autoinjector of pralidoxime chloride (600 mg). Each soldier is issued three ATNAAs (Figure 4-1).

Diazepam is an anticonvulsant drug used to decrease convulsive activity and reduce the brain damage caused by prolonged seizure activity. Without the use of pyridostigmine pretreatment, experimental animals died quickly after superlethal doses of nerve agents despite conventional therapy. With pyridostigmine pretreatment (followed by conventional therapy), animals survived superlethal doses of soman but had prolonged periods of seizure activity before recovery. They later

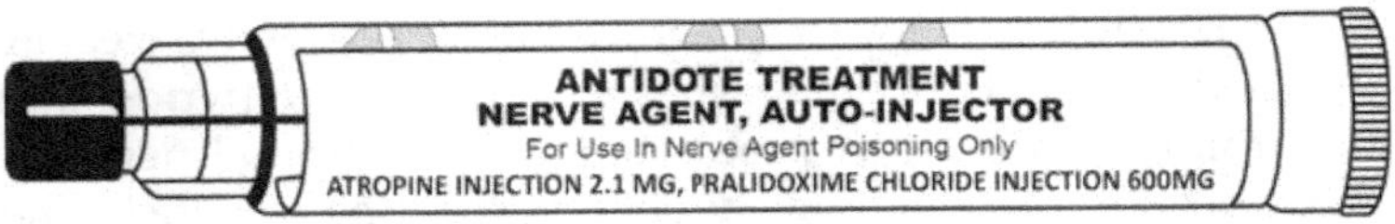

Figure 4-1. Antidote Treatment Nerve Agent Autoinjector (ATNAA).

had performance decrements and anatomic lesions in their brains. The administration of diazepam with other standard therapy to soman-exposed animals pretreated with pyridostigmine reduced the seizure activity and its sequelae. Current military doctrine is to administer diazepam with other therapy (three ATNAAs) at the onset of severe effects from a nerve agent, whether or not seizure activity is among those effects. In addition to the other autoinjectors, each soldier carries an autoinjector containing 10 mg of diazepam for administration by a buddy (soldiers who are able to self-administer would not need it). *Diazepam should be given if administration of three ATNAAs is required***.** Medical personnel can administer more diazepam to a casualty if necessary. Medics may carry extra diazepam injectors (Figure 4-2) and are authorized to administer two additional injectors at 10-minute intervals to a convulsing casualty. (**NOTE:** Midazolam will replace diazepam in the CANA in the near future.)

The doctrine for *self-aid* for nerve agent intoxication states that if an individual has effects from the agent, one ATNAA should be self-administered. If there is no improvement in 10 minutes, a buddy should be sought to assist in the evaluation of the soldier's condition before further ATNAAs are given. If

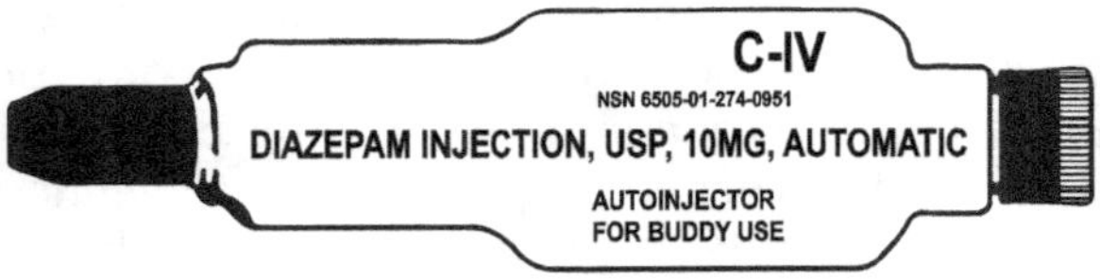

Figure 4-2. Convulsive Antidote, Nerve Agent (CANA) autoinjector.

a buddy finds an individual severely intoxicated (eg, gasping respiration, twitching) so he or she cannot self-administer an ATNAA, the buddy should administer three ATNAAs and diazepam immediately (Figures 4-3–4-6). The discussion below is advice for medical assistance.

The appropriate number of ATNAAs to administer initially to a nerve agent vapor casualty depends on the severity of effects. Systemic atropine will not reverse miosis (unless administered in very large amounts), and miosis alone is not an indication for an ATNAA. If the eye or head pain and nausea associated with miosis are severe, topical application of atropine (or homatropine) in the eye will bring relief. Topical atropine should not be used without good reason (severe pain), because it causes blurred vision for a day or longer. A casualty with miosis and rhinorrhea should be given one ATNAA only if the rhinorrhea is severe and troublesome (preventing the soldier from wearing a mask because of fluid). A casualty with mild to moderate dyspnea should be given one or two ATNAAs, depending on the severity of distress and the time between exposure and therapy. Respiratory distress

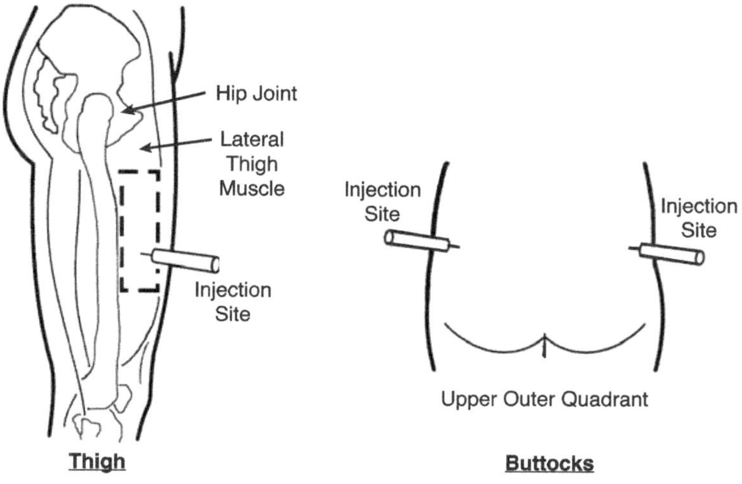

Figure 4-3. Primary (thigh) and secondary (buttocks) injection sites.

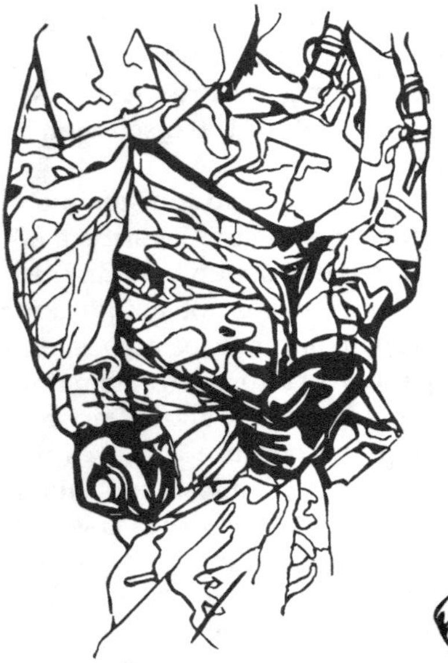

Figure 4-4. Self-aid injection.

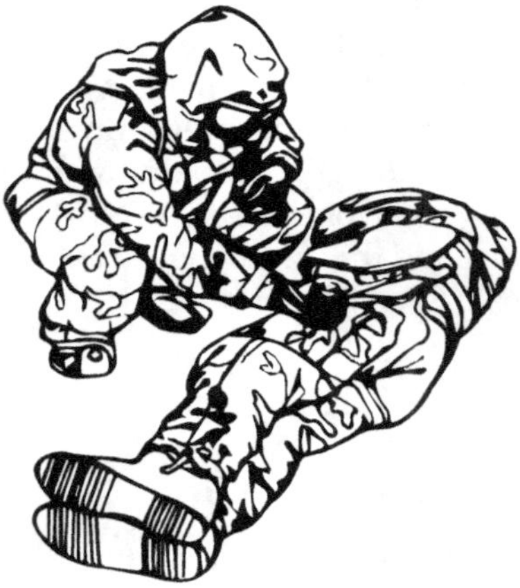

Figure 4-5. Buddy-aid injection.

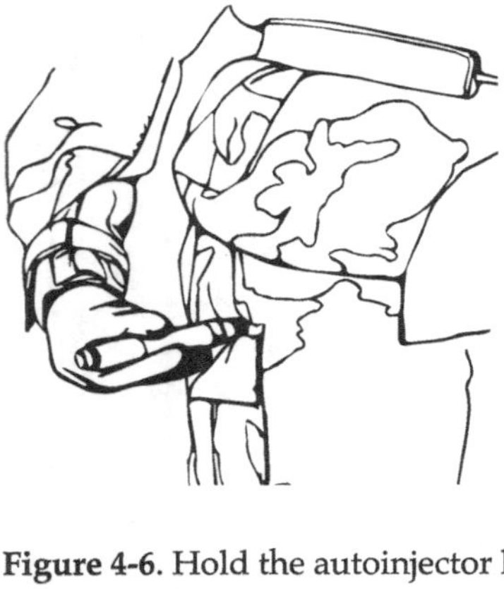

Figure 4-6. Hold the autoinjector like a pen.

from a mild exposure will spontaneously decrease within 15 to 30 minutes after termination of exposure, so if the casualty is not severely uncomfortable, only one ATNAA should be used initially. Atropine is quite effective, and care should be taken not to give too much to a casualty who does not need it.

A severe casualty of nerve agent vapor has miosis, copious secretions from the nose and mouth, severe difficulty breathing or apnea, possibly some degree of cyanosis, muscular fasciculations, and twitching or convulsive activity, and is unconscious. He or she should be given three ATNAAs and diazepam immediately. Ventilation will be needed and should be done via an endotracheal airway if possible. Suctioning of excessive airway secretions will be necessary to enhance air exchange and will make ventilatory efforts easier. Administration of atropine, in 2-mg doses, should be repeated at 3- to 5-minute intervals and should be titrated to a reduction of secretions and reduction of ventilatory resistance. When the IV preparation is available, the preferred route of atropine administration is via the IV route, but this route should be avoided until hypoxia is corrected, because intravenously administered atropine in hypoxic animals has produced ventricular fibrillation. In a hypotensive patient or a patient with tenuous venous access, atropine might be given intratracheally, either via the endotracheal tube or directly into the trachea, for more rapid absorption via the peribronchial vessels.

The medical care provider might overestimate the required atropine use in a mild to moderate casualty. More importantly, the care provider might underestimate atropine dosing by administering too little to a severe casualty. In a severe casualty, atropine should be pushed at frequent intervals until secretions are dry (or nearly dry) and until ventilation can be accomplished with ease. In reported cases this has required 10 to 20 mg of atropine within the first several hours. A conscious, less severely exposed casualty should receive atropine until breathing comfortably, and able to communicate this. Dry secretions need not be an endpoint in mild to moderate casualties.

The casualty with skin exposure to liquid is more difficult to evaluate and manage than is a vapor exposure casualty. Agent on the surface of the skin can be decontaminated, but agent absorbed into the skin cannot be removed. The initial effects from absorbed liquid agent can start 2 to 3 hours after thorough decontamination of agent droplets on the skin. A casualty from liquid exposure on the skin may continue to worsen because of continued absorption of the agent from the skin depot.

The first effects of a liquid droplet on the skin are sweating with or without blanching, and occasionally muscular fasciculations at the site. GI effects (nausea, vomiting, and sometimes diarrhea) are the first systemic effects, and these may start from 0.5 to 18 hours after contact with the agent. If these effects occur within the first several hours after exposure, they may portend more severe effects, and initial therapy should be two ATNAAs. If effects begin later, initial therapy should be one ATNAA.

A large amount of liquid agent on the skin will cause effects 1 to 30 minutes after contact, whether or not decontamination was done. Nevertheless, early decontamination may lessen the magnitude of the effects. After the latent or asymptomatic period, the casualty will suddenly lose consciousness and begin seizure activity. The condition of the casualty and management are the same as described for a severe casualty of vapor exposure.

Further care of the severe casualty consists of atropine administration to minimize secretions and ventilation until spontaneous respiration resumes. Oxime administration should be repeated at hourly intervals for two or three additional doses. The preferred method of administration of the oxime is by IV drip of 1 g over 20 to 30 minutes (more rapid administration will cause hypertension), but three additional oxime autoinjectors (a total dose of 1.8 grams) may be given if the IV route cannot be used. The need for ventilation may continue for 0.5 to 3 hours. Unless prolonged hypoxia or other complications have occurred, the casualty will eventually begin having spontaneous muscular activity and make sporadic attempts to breathe. Muscles will become stronger and breathing more regular, and the casualty will have intermittent episodes of conscious behavior. Within an hour or two, these casualties will be breathing, moving, and conscious, although they will be weak and intermittently obtunded.

Pretreatment

In late 1990s, the US military fielded pyridostigmine bromide as a pretreatment for nerve agent exposure. Each service member received a blister pack containing 21 30-mg tablets. The dose regimen is one 30-mg tablet every 8 hours. When to start and stop dosing is a division or corps' command decision, made with the advice of the intelligence, chemical, and medical staffs, and not a local decision or individual decision. Thus, pyridostigmine is, in a sense, not a medical treatment but a defensive weapons system.

Pyridostigmine bromide is the drug of choice for myasthenia gravis and has been approved for the treatment of this disease since 1951. In 2003 the US Food and Drug Administration approved additional on-label use of pyridostigmine bromide for pretreatment against soman. Consequently, commanders have the authority to order its use without service members' consent, exactly as they may order an approved vaccine.

Pyridostigmine is pretreatment, *not* an antidote. It should be taken before soman exposure. It is ineffective unless standard ATNAA therapy is also used in the appropriate manner. When given before soman exposure and when that exposure is followed by the standard ATNAA therapy, pretreatment increases the LD_{50} several fold over the LD_{50} that occurs without the use of the pretreatment. Functionally, this means that a soldier can survive what would otherwise have been a lethal dose; instead of dying, the casualty is a very sick patient who can be saved when antidotes are properly and promptly administered. When soman is the nerve agent, the use of pyridostigmine increases survival. When the agent is GB or VX, survival after standard ATNAA therapy is essentially the same whether or not pyridostigmine pretreatment is used; that is, pyridostigmine use provides no benefit in GB or VX poisoning. Current data are not adequate to evaluate the effectiveness of pyridostigmine pretreatment for GA or GF exposure.One consequence of the greater survival from the use of pyridostigmine is prolonged seizure activity and subsequent possible brain damage in the survivors. The early administration of diazepam will decrease these effects.

In the 1960s, it was noted that carbamates bind to the active site of cholinesterase in a similar manner as the binding of organophosphonate cholinesterase inhibitors to cholinesterase. Additionally, while the carbamate is attached to the active site, an organophosphorus compound can not attach to the enzyme. The carbamate-enzyme binding, or carbamoylation, lasts only for hours, rather than for the lifetime of the enzyme as does the organophosphorus compound attachment, and is therefore spontaneously reversible. While the enzyme is carbamoylated, the active site is protected from attack by other compounds such as organophosphorus cholinesterase inhibitors, including nerve agents. After several hours, the carbamate leaves the enzyme (ie, decarbamoylation occurs), and the enzyme becomes completely functional again. Thus, the carbamate provides temporary protection for the enzyme against nerve agent attack. People have far more acetylcholinesterase than they need, so the use of pyridostigmine to carbamoylate a small proportion of acetylcholinesterase converts that proportion into a reserve that will be available to save the patient if soman attack inactivates the rest.

Many carbamates have been investigated for their effectiveness and their safety. Pyridostigmine was found effective and underwent extensive testing in humans. It has a 45-year safety record and is used by over 16,000 myasthenic patients in the United States on a daily basis. Investigations indicated that it did not interfere with the performance of military tasks and caused no adverse physiological disturbances.

Tens of thousands of US troops took pyridostigmine during the Persian Gulf War. The incidence of side effects (primarily GI and urinary) was over 50%, but only a few percent of the troops sought medical care for severity of these effects. Medical officers discontinued the drug in less than 1% of cases.

Triage

A severe nerve agent casualty who is unconscious, convulsing or postictal, breathing with difficulty or apneic, and possibly flaccid will survive with appropriate, immediate therapy, including ventilation, if circulation is intact. This casualty should be triaged as *immediate* if therapy can be provided. If a blood pressure cannot be obtained, the casualty may be considered *expectant*.

Casualties with severe symptoms who are spontaneously breathing, have not lost consciousness, and have not seized have an excellent chance of survival with a minimal amount of therapeutic effort. They should be categorized as *immediate* and given three ATNAAs and diazepam. The casualty may worsen if exposure was to liquid, and atropine administration should be repeated. If the casualty loses consciousness, seizes, and becomes apneic, retriage and administer further care based on available resources.

Casualties who are walking and talking and are no longer being exposed to agent will usually be triaged as *minimal*. If a casualty can walk and talk, then breathing and circulation are intact. There is no indication for immediate life-saving care. This does not preclude self-administration or medic administration of additional antidote for symptoms.

A casualty recovering from a severe exposure who has received large doses of antidotes and has been ventilated will be triaged as *delayed* for further medical observation or care. A casualty who suffered liquid exposure and has been both treated and decontaminated may also be triaged as delayed.

Return to Duty

Return to duty depends on the status of the casualty, his or her assignment, and the tactical situation. Studies indicate that animals with decreased erythrocyte acetylcholinesterase activity from a nerve agent exposure have a decreased LD_{50} for another nerve agent exposure (they are more susceptible to the agent) until that cholinesterase activity returns to at least 75% of its baseline, or to preexposure activity. Nerve agent-exposed workers in a depot or research facility are prevented from returning to work with agents until this recovery occurs. In a battlefield situation, conservative management should be balanced against the mission and the risk of repeated exposure to a large amount of agent.

In a military field situation, the capability to analyze blood for erythrocyte cholinesterase activity is usually not available, and the baseline activity of each individual is not known. The erythrocyte cholinesterase activity in a casualty with severe systemic effects will be inhibited by 70% or greater (30% or less of preexposure activity), and 45 days or longer will be required for cholinesterase activity to return to 75% of preexposure activity. The enzyme activity of a casualty with mild or moderate effects from agent vapor may be nearly normal or may be markedly inhibited. Predictions of erythrocyte cholinesterase recovery time are unreliable.

Most individuals triaged as minimal may return to duty within hours if the mission requires these personnel, although lingering ocular and CNS effects may be limiting factors in these cases. These individuals may be able to fire a rifle, but their performance might be decremented because of both visual problems and difficulty in concentrating. These prolonged effects must be evaluated before the casualties return to duty.

Casualties who had severe effects might be walking and talking after 6 to 24 hours but may be unfit for most duties. Ideally, they should be kept under medical observation for a week or longer and not returned to duty until recovery of cholinesterase activity. However, the mission may lead to modification of these guidelines.

Long-Term Effects

Minor electroencephalographic (EEG) changes were noted more than a year after nerve agent exposure when averaged EEGs in a group of individauls exposed to a nerve agent were compared to a control group. EEG changes could not be identified in individuals. Neuropsychiatric pathologies have been noted in individuals for weeks to months after exposure to insecticides. Both in the Tokyo subway attack and in the Iran-Iraq War, reports of long-term neuropsychiatric changes after exposure to nerve agent have surfaced. Little is known about the pathophysiology of these syndromes. They are not dose-related and do overlap with posttraumatic stress disorder.

Polyneuropathy, reported after organophosphate insecticide poisoning, has not been reported in humans exposed to nerve agents and has been produced in animals only at unsurvivable doses. The intermediate syndrome has not been reported in humans after nerve agent exposure, nor has it been produced in animals. Muscular necrosis has occurred in animals after high-dose nerve agent exposure but reversed within weeks; it has not been reported in humans.

Chapter 5

INCAPACITATING AGENTS

Summary

NATO Code: BZ

Signs and Symptoms: Mydriasis; dry mouth; dry skin; increased deep tendon reflexes; decreased level of consciousness; confusion; disorientation; disturbances in perception and interpretation (illusions and/or hallucinations); denial of illness; short attention span; impaired memory.

Field Detection: No field detector is available.

Decontamination: Gentle but thorough flushing of skin and hair with water or soap and water is all that is required. Remove clothing.

Management: Antidote: physostigmine. *Supportive:* monitoring of vital signs, especially core temperature.

Overview

BZ, or 3-quinuclidinyl benzilate, is a glycolate anticholinergic compound dispersed as an aerosolized solid when intended for inhalation, or as agent dissolved in one or more solvents when intended for ingestion or percutaneous absorption. Acting as a competitive inhibitor of acetylcholine at postsynaptic and postjunctional muscarinic receptor sites, BZ causes peripheral nervous system (PNS) effects that in general are the opposite of those seen in nerve agent poisoning. Central nervous system

(CNS) effects include stupor, confusion, and confabulation with concrete and panoramic illusions and hallucinations, and with regression to automatic "phantom" behaviors such as plucking and disrobing. The combination of anticholinergic PNS and CNS effects aids in the diagnosis of patients exposed to these agents. Physostigmine, which increases the concentration of acetylcholine in synapses and in neuromuscular and neuroglandular junctions, is a specific antidote.

History and Military Relevance

The use of chemicals to induce altered states of mind dates to antiquity and includes the use of plants such as thorn apple (*Datura stramonium*) that contain combinations of anticholinergic alkaloids. The use of nonlethal chemicals to render an enemy force incapable of fighting dates back to ancient Greece, where, according to some accounts, in 600 BCE Solon's soldiers threw hellebore roots into streams supplying water to enemy troops, who then developed diarrhea. In 184 BCE Hannibal's army used belladonna plants to induce disorientation, and in AD 1672 the Bishop of Muenster attempted to use belladonna-containing grenades in an assault on the city of Groningen. In 1881, members of a railway surveying expedition crossing Tuareg territory in North Africa ate dried dates that tribesmen had apparently deliberately contaminated with *Hyoscyamus falezlez*, causing intoxication, excruciating pain, weakness, and unintelligible speech. In 1908, 200 French soldiers in Hanoi became delirious and experienced hallucinations after being poisoned with a related plant. More recently, Soviet use of incapacitating agents internally and in Afghanistan was alleged, but never substantiated.

Following World War II, the US military investigated a wide range of possible nonlethal, psychobehavioral, chemical incapacitating agents including psychedelic indoles such as lysergic acid diethylamide (LSD-25) and marijuana derivatives, certain tranquilizers, and several glycolate anticholinergics. BZ was one of the anticholinergic compounds. It was weaponized beginning in the 1960s for possible battlefield use. Although BZ figured prominently in the plot of the 1990 movie *Jacob's Ladder* as the compound responsible for hallucinations and violent deaths in a fictitious American battalion in Vietnam, this agent never saw operational use. Destruction of American stockpiles began in 1988 and is now complete.

In February 1998, the British Ministry of Defence released an intelligence report that accused Iraq of having stockpiled large amounts of a glycolate anticholinergic incapacitating agent known as Agent 15. This compound is speculated either to be identical to BZ or a closely related derivative. Also in 1998, there were allegations that elements of the Yugoslav People's Army used incapacitating agents that caused hallucinations and irrational behavior against fleeing Bosnian refugees. Physical evidence of BZ use in Bosnia remains elusive, however.

Nomenclature

The term "incapacitation," when used in a general sense, is roughly equivalent to the term "disability" as used in occupational medicine and denotes the inability to perform a task because of a quantifiable physical or mental impairment. In this sense, any of the chemical warfare agents may incapacitate a victim; however, again by the military definition of this type of agent, incapacitation refers to impairments that are temporary and nonlethal. Thus, riot-control agents are incapacitating because they cause temporary loss of vision due to blepharospasm, but they are not considered military incapacitants because the loss of vision does not last long.

Although incapacitation may result from physiological changes such as mucous membrane irritation, diarrhea, or hyperthermia, the term "incapacitating agent" as militarily defined refers to a compound that produces temporary and nonlethal impairment of military performance by virtue of its psychobehavioral or CNS effects.

Nonmilitary Sources

BZ and related anticholinergic compounds can be synthesized in clandestine laboratories, but their illicit use is uncommon, possibly because of some unpleasant effects such as dry mouth and skin. The anticholinergics atropine, oxybutynin, and scopolamine find use in clinical medicine and are available as pharmaceuticals, as are antihistamines that have prominent anticholinergic side effects. BZ is widely used in pharmacology as a muscarinic receptor marker. As mentioned above, anticholinergic hallucinogenic compounds are present in thorn apple as well as other plants of the family *Solanaceae*, which also includes black henbane (*Hyoscyamus niger*), belladonna (or deadly nightshade, *Atropa belladonna*), woody nightshade (*Solanum dulcamara*), and Jerusalem cherry (*Solanum pseudocapsicum*). These plants contain varying proportions of the anticholinergic glycolates atropine, hyoscyamine, and hyoscine.

Physiochemical Characteristics

BZ is odorless. It is stable in most solvents, with a half-life of 3 to 4 weeks in moist air; even heat-producing munitions can disperse it. It is extremely persistent in soil and water and on most surfaces. It is also soluble in propylene glycol, dimethyl sulfoxide, and other solvents. Agent 15 presumably shares many of the physiochemical properties of BZ.

Detection and Protection

Because BZ is odorless and nonirritating, and because clinical effects are not seen until after a latent period of 30 minutes to 24 hours, exposure could occur without the knowledge of casualties. No currently available field military or civilian detector is designed to disclose the presence of BZ or other anticholinergic compounds in the environment. Confirmation of the exact chemical involved in an incapacitating agent exposure requires laboratory analysis of environmental specimens containing the agent. The high-efficiency particulate air (HEPA) filter in the canister of the chemical protective mask prevents exposure of the face and respiratory tract to aerosolized BZ. The chemical protective ensemble protects the skin against contact with BZ or other incapacitating agents dispersed as fine solid particles or in solution. Protection against ingestion would depend upon a high index of suspicion for BZ-contaminated food or drink.

Toxicokinetics

Bioavailability of BZ via ingestion and by inhalation of 1-μm particles approximates 80% and 40% to 50%, respectively. Percutaneous absorption of BZ dissolved in propylene glycol yields, after a latent period of up to 24 hours, serum levels approximately 5% to 10% of those achieved with intravenous (IV) or intramuscular (IM) administration. Although inhalation of aerosolized BZ is probably the greatest risk on the battlefield, terrorists may choose to disseminate BZ in forms that provide significant opportunities for ingestion and absorption through the skin.

Following absorption, BZ is systemically distributed to most organs and tissues of the body. Its ability to reach synapses and neuromuscular and neuroglandular junctions throughout the body is responsible for its PNS effects, whereas its ability to cross the blood-brain barrier is responsible for its CNS effects. Atropine and hyoscyamine both cross the placenta and can be found in small quantities in breast milk; whether this is also true for BZ is unclear. Metabolism of BZ occurs primarily in the liver, with elimination of unchanged agent and metabolites chiefly in the urine.

Toxicity

The characteristic that makes BZ and other glycolates an incapacitating rather than a toxic chemical warfare agent is its high safety ratio. The amount required to produce effects is a thousand or more times less than a fatal dose of the compound. The ICt_{50} (the concentration-time product needed to produce incapacitation in 50% of an exposed group) for BZ is 112 mg•min/m^3, whereas the LCt_{50} (median lethal concentration) is estimated to be almost 2,000 times the dose needed for incapacitation.

Mechanism of Action

The agent BZ and other anticholinergic glycolates act as competitive inhibitors of the neurotransmitter acetylcholine neurons at two places: (1) postjunctional muscarinic receptors in cardiac and smooth muscle and in exocrine (ducted) glands and (2) postsynaptic receptors in neurons. As the concentration of BZ at these sites increases, the proportion of receptors available for binding to acetylcholine decreases, and the end organ "sees" less acetylcholine. (One way of visualizing this process is to imagine BZ coating the surface of the end organ and preventing acetylcholine from reaching its receptors.) Because BZ has little to no agonist activity with respect to acetylcholine, high concentrations of BZ essentially block acetylcholine at these sites, leading to clinical effects reflective of understimulation of end organs.

Clinical Effects

Peripheral Effects

- Mydriasis, blurred vision
- Dry mouth, dry skin
- Initially rapid heart rate; later, normal or slow heart rate
- Possible atropine flush

The PNS effects of BZ are, in general, readily understood as those of understimulation of end organs and are qualitatively similar to those of atropine. Due to PNS effects, patients have been described as "dry as a bone, hot as a hare, red as a beet, and blind as a bat." Decreased stimulation of eccrine and apocrine sweat glands in the skin results in dry skin and a reduction in the ability to dissipate heat by evaporative cooling. The skin becomes warm partly from decreased sweating and partly from compensatory cutaneous vasodilatation (the skin becomes red, with a so-called atropine flush) as the body attempts to shunt a higher proportion of core-temperature blood as close as possible to the surface of the skin. With heat loss decreased, the core temperature itself rises. Understimulation of other exocrine glands leads to dry mouth, thirst, and decreased secretions from lacrimal, nasal, bronchial, and gastrointestinal glands.

Decreased cholinergic stimulation of pupillary sphincter muscles allows α-adrenergically innervated pupillary dilating muscles to act essentially unopposed, resulting in mydriasis.

(In fact, the cosmetic effect of mydriasis in women who applied extracts of deadly nightshade topically to their eyes explains the name "belladonna" [beautiful lady] given to this plant.) Similar effects on cholinergic ciliary muscles produce paralysis of accommodation. Other smooth muscle effects from BZ intoxication include decreased bladder tone and decreased urinary force with possibly severe bladder distention.

Typically BZ initially raises the heart rate, but hours later, depending on the dose of BZ, the heart rate returns to baseline or may become bradycardic. Either the peripheral vagal blockade has ceased, or the stimulation of the vagal nucleus has occurred.

Neither atropine nor BZ can act directly at the postjunctional nicotinic receptors found in skeletal muscle, but BZ-exposed patients nonetheless exhibit muscle weakness. This weakness, along with incoordination, heightened stretch reflexes, and ataxia, is probably due to the effects of BZ at CNS sites.

Central Effects

- Disturbances in level of consciousness
- Misperceptions and difficulty in interpretation (delusions, hallucinations)
- Poor judgment and insight (illness denial)
- Short attention span, distractibility, impaired memory (particularly recent)
- Slurred speech, perseveration
- Disorientation
- Ataxia
- Variability (quiet/restless)

The PNS effects of BZ are essentially side effects that are useful in diagnosis but incidental to the CNS effects for which the incapacitating agents were developed. These CNS effects include a dose-dependent decrease in the level of consciousness, beginning with drowsiness and progressing through sedation to stupor and coma. The patient is often disoriented to time and place. Disturbances in judgment and insight occur. The patient may abandon socially imposed restraints and resort to vulgar and inappropriate behavior. Perceptual clues may no longer be readily interpretable. The patient is easily distracted and may have memory loss, most notably short-term memory. In the face of these deficits, patients try to make sense of their environment and will not hesitate to make up answers on the spot to questions that confuse them. Speech becomes slurred and often senseless, and loss of inflection produces a flat, monotonous voice. References become concrete and semiautomatic, with colloquialisms, clichés, profanity, and perseveration. Handwriting also deteriorates. Semiautomatic behavior may also include disrobing (perhaps partly because of increased body temperature), mumbling, and phantom behaviors such as constant picking, plucking, or grasping motions ("woolgathering" or carphology).

CNS-mediated perceptual disturbances in BZ poisoning include both illusions (misidentification of real objects) and hallucinations (the perception of objects or attributes that have no objective reality). (Although the phrase "mad as a hatter" refers to poisoning from mercury formerly used by hatters on felt, it can just as well serve as a reminder of CNS effects from anticholinergics.) Anticholinergic hallucinations differ from the often vague, ineffable, and often transcendent-appearing hallucinations induced by hallucinogenic indoles such as LSD. Hallucinations from BZ tend to be realistic, distinct, easily identifiable (often commonly encountered objects or persons), and panoramic, and they usually become less extreme during the course of the intoxication.

Another prominent CNS finding in BZ poisoning is behavioral lability, with patients swinging back and forth between quiet confusion and self-absorption in hallucinations to frank combativeness. Moreover, as other symptoms begin to resolve, intermittent paranoia may be seen. Automatic behaviors common during resolution include the crawling or climbing motions called "progresso obstinato" in old descriptions of dementia.

BZ produces effects not just in individuals, but also in groups, with shared illusions and hallucinations (*folie à deux, folie en famille,* and "mass hysteria"). For example, two BZ-intoxicated individuals took turns smoking an imaginary cigarette clearly visible to both of them but to no one else.

Time Course of Effects

Clinical effects from ingestion or inhalation of BZ appear after an asymptomatic or latent period that may be as little as 30 minutes or as long as 24 hours; the usual range is 30 minutes to 4 hours, with a mean of 2 hours. However, effects may not appear up to 36 hours after skin exposure to BZ. Once effects appear, their duration is typically 72 to 96 hours and dose-dependent. Following an ICt_{50} of BZ, severe effects may last 36 hours, but mild effects may persist for an additional day.

The clinical course from BZ poisoning can be divided into the following four stages:

1. Onset or induction (0 to 4 hours after exposure), characterized by parasympathetic blockade and mild CNS effects.
2. Second phase (4 to 20 hours after exposure), characterized by stupor with ataxia and hyperthermia.
3. Third phase (20 to 96 hours after exposure), in which full-blown delirium is seen but often fluctuates from moment to moment.
4. Fourth phase, or resolution, characterized by paranoia, deep sleep, reawakening, crawling or climbing automatisms, and eventual reorientation.

Differential Diagnosis

The differential diagnosis for irrational and confused patients is a long one (Table 5-1) and includes anxiety reactions as well as intoxication with a variety of agents, including hallucinogenic indoles (such as LSD), cannabinoids (such as the δ-9-tetrahydrocannabinol in marijuana), lead, barbiturates, and bromides. All of these conditions can lead to restlessness, lightheadedness (with associated vertigo and ataxia), confusion, and erratic behavior, with or without vomiting. Clues that specifically point to BZ or a related compound are the combination of anticholinergic PNS effects ("dry as a bone, hot as a hare, red as a beet, and blind as a bat") with the CNS effects ("mad as a hatter") of slurred and monotonous speech, automatic behavior (perseveration, disrobing, and phantom

Table 5-1. Differential Diagnosis for Incapacitating Agent Exposure

Signs and Symptoms	Possible Etiology
Restlessness, dizziness, or giddiness; failure to obey orders, confusion, erratic behavior; stumbling or staggering; vomiting.	Anticholinergics, indoles (LSD), cannabinols, anxiety reaction, other intoxicants (alcohol, lead, bromides, barbiturates).
Dry mouth, tachycardia at rest, elevated temperature, facial flushing, blurred vision, pupillary dilation, slurred or nonsensical speech, hallucinatory behavior, disrobing, mumbling and picking behavior, stupor and coma.	Anticholinergics
Inappropriate smiling or laughter, irrational fear, difficulty expressing self, distractibility, perceptual distortions, labile increase in pupil size, increased heart rate and blood pressure, stomach cramps, vomiting.	Indoles (Schizophrenic psychosis may mimic these symptoms in some respects.)
Euphoric, relaxed, unconcerned attitude; daydreaming; easy laughter; hypotension and dizziness on sudden standing.	Cannabinols
Tremor, clinging or pleading, crying, clear answers, phobias, decrease in disturbance with reassurance, history of nervousness or immaturity.	Anxiety reaction

LSD: lysergic acid diethylamide

behaviors ["woolgathering"]), and vivid, realistic, describable hallucinations (decreasing in size over time) in a patient slipping into and out of delirium.

Atropine intoxication from autoinjector use in a patient not exposed to nerve agents may create similar PNS effects to those seen in BZ intoxication. However, marked confusion from atropine is not normally seen until a total of six or seven autoinjectors have been given (in a hot, dehydrated, or battle-stressed individual, less atropine would probably suffice). Circumstantial evidence may be helpful in differential diagnosis.

Heat stroke may also generate hot, dry, and confused or stuporous casualties and must be considered. Patients with anxiety reactions are usually oriented to time, place, and person but may be trembling, crying, or otherwise panicked. The classic picture of unconcern may characterize a patient with a conversion reaction, but these patients are also likely to be oriented and lack the anticholinergic PNS signs of BZ poisoning.

Medical Management

These guidelines for general patient care are not intended to take the place of sound clinical judgment, especially in the management of complicated cases. The admonition to protect oneself first may be difficult when dealing with any intoxication involving a latent period, since healthcare providers may already have been exposed during the same time frame as patients. Protection of medical staff from BZ that has already been absorbed and systemically distributed in a patient is not needed.

General supportive management of the patient includes decontamination of skin and clothing (ineffective for agent that has already been absorbed but useful in preventing further absorption of any agent still in contact with the patient), confiscation of weapons and related items from the patient, and observation. Physical restraint may be required in moderately to severely affected patients. The greatest risks to the patient's life are (*a*) injuries from his or her own erratic behavior (or from the behavior of similarly intoxicated patients) and (*b*) hyperthermia, especially in patients who are in hot or humid environments or are dehydrated from overexertion or insufficient water intake. A severely exposed patient may be comatose with serious cardiac arrhythmias and electrolyte disturbances. Managing heat stress is a high priority in these patients. Because of the prolonged time course in BZ poisoning, consideration should always be given to evacuation to a higher care level.

Because BZ effectively decreases the amount of acetylcholine "seen" by postsynaptic and postjunctional receptors, specific antidotal therapy in BZ poisoning is geared toward raising the concentration of acetylcholine in these synapses and junctions. Any compound that causes a rise in acetylcholine concentration can potentially overcome BZ-induced inhibition and restore normal functioning; even the nerve agent VX has been shown to be effective when given under carefully controlled conditions. The specific antidote of choice in BZ poisoning is the carbamate anticholinesterase physostigmine, which temporarily raises acetylcholine concentrations by binding reversibly to anticholinesterase on the postsynaptic or postjunctional membrane. Physostigmine is similar in many ways to pyridostigmine and is equally effective when used as a preexposure antidotal enhancer (pretreatment) in individuals at high risk for subsequently encountering soman. However, physostigmine is not used for this purpose because the doses required cause vomiting through CNS mechanisms. In the case of BZ poisoning, a nonpolar compound such as physostigmine is used specifically because penetration into the brain is required in those individuals who already have CNS effects from BZ.

In BZ-intoxicated patients, physostigmine is minimally effective during the first 4 hours after exposure but is very effective after 4 hours. Oral dosing generally requires one and a half times the amount of antidote as does IM or IV administration. However, effects from a single intramuscular injection of physostigmine last only about 60 minutes, necessitating frequent re-dosing. It must be emphasized that physostigmine does not shorten the clinical course of BZ poisoning and that relapses will occur if treatment is discontinued prematurely. The temptation to substitute a slow IV infusion for IM injections should be tempered by the awareness that IV infusion may lead to bradycardia (similar to that caused by nerve agents), and too rapid infusion can cause arrhythmias, excessive secretions (to the point of compromising air exchange), and convulsions. Moreover, the sodium bisulfite in commercially available preparations of physostigmine may cause life-threatening allergic responses.

Suggested Dosages of Physostigmine

- **Test dose.** If the diagnosis is in doubt, a dose of 1 mg may be given. If a slight improvement occurs, routine dosing should be given.

- **Routine dosing.** Adult doses of about 45 μg/kg have been recommended, which may be modified by the response. A mental status examination should be done every hour, and the dose and time interval of dosing should be modified according to whether or not mental status is improved. As the patient improves, the dosage requirement will decrease. Oral dosing is the preferred route after the initial IV dose. This will decrease the risk of overdose that could be created by further IV administration.
- **Routes of administration**. For each route, titrate about every 60 minutes to mental status.
  - IM: 45 μg/kg in adults (20 mg/kg in children)
  - IV: 30 μg/kg slowly (1 mg/min)
  - PO (by mouth): 60 μg/kg if patient is cooperative (because of bitter taste, consider diluting in juice)

History and Toxicity of Physostigmine

The antagonism between physostigmine (derived from the calabar bean) and atropine (tincture of belladonna) was first reported in 1864 by a physician who successfully treated prisoners who had become delirious after drinking tincture of belladonna. Physicians did not notice this report until the 1950s, when atropine coma (in which 50 mg or so of atropine was given to certain psychiatric patients) was successfully treated with physostigmine after the "therapeutic benefit" had been attained. Again, this went unnoticed until a controlled study reported in 1967 indicated that anticholinergic intoxication could be successfully, albeit transiently, reversed by physostigmine.

The administration of physostigmine by the IV route in a delirious but conscious and otherwise healthy patient is not without peril. It is sometimes difficult to keep a delirious patient quiet long enough to administer the drug. Even if administered correctly (very slowly), the heart rate may decline from 110 to 45 beats per minute over a period of 1 to 2 minutes. The difference in the onset of the effects after IM and IV administration of physostigmine is a matter of only several minutes. Since its use is rarely lifesaving, this slight difference in time of response is inconsequential. Refer to the product insert for dosage and administration.

Physostigmine is a safe and effective antidote if used properly. In a conscious and delirious patient it will produce very effective but transient reversal of both the peripheral and central effects of cholinergic-blocking compounds. Its use by the IV route is not without hazards. It should NOT be used in a patient with cardiorespiratory compromise, hypoxia, or acid-base imbalance with a history of seizure disorders or arrhythmias.

Triage

A casualty with cardiorespiratory compromise or severe hyperthermia should be considered *immediate*. Casualties in this condition are possible, though unlikely. Immediate attention to ventilation, hemodynamic status, and temperature control may be lifesaving. Because of its dangers in a hypoxic or hemodynamically challenged patient, physostigmine should be considered a second-line management option to be used only if adequate attention can simultaneously be given to temperature and other vital signs.

A casualty with pronounced or worsening anticholinergic signs should be triaged as *delayed*, and physostigmine should be considered.

A casualty with mild PNS or CNS anticholinergic effects may be considered *minimal*. Given the time course of BZ intoxication, however, these patients should not be considered able to manage themselves or capable of routine return to duty, and should be relieved of their weapons, observed, and if the holding capacity at the current role is exceeded, evacuated.

A casualty with severe cardiorespiratory compromise when treatment or evacuation resources are insufficient may be considered *expectant*; however, patients in this condition are also unlikely.

Return to Duty

Given the time course of the intoxication, early return to duty is probably not a realistic possibility for the majority of casualties, who may require observation and management for at least several days.

Chapter 6

RIOT-CONTROL AGENTS

Summary

NATO Codes: CS, CN, CR, DM, and OC

Signs and Symptoms: Burning and pain on exposed mucous membranes and skin, eye pain and tearing, burning in the nostrils, respiratory discomfort, and tingling of the exposed skin. DM causes prolonged periods of vomiting and a feeling of malaise.

Field Detection: No field detector is available for any of the riot-contral agents.

Decontamination: Eyes: Thoroughly flush with water, saline, or similar substance. *Skin (CS, CN, CR, and DM)*: Flush with copious amounts of water, soap and water, or a mildly alkaline solution (sodium bicarbonate or sodium carbonate). Generally, decontamination is not needed if the wind is brisk. *Skin (OC):* The pain from OC will increase with water, especially warm water. It is best decontaminated with baby shampoo, milk, alcohol, or vegetable oil. Without decontamination pain will subside over time.

Management: Usually none is necessary; effects are self-limiting and diminish or cease within 45 minutes. DM is the exception; its effects may last several hours.

Overview

Riot-control agents, also called irritants, lacrimators, and tear gas, produce transient discomfort and eye closure, rendering the recipient temporarily incapable of fighting or resisting. Law enforcement agencies use them for riot control, and military forces use them for training and in combat. They have a high median lethal concentration (LCt_{50}) and a low median effective concentration (ECt_{50}), and therefore a high safety ratio. Their major effect is to cause pain, burning, or discomfort on exposed mucous membranes and skin; these effects occur within seconds of exposure but seldom persist more than a few minutes after exposure has ended.

History and Military Relevance

Paris police used riot-control agents to dispel rioters before World War I, and these compounds were the first chemical agents deployed during that war. French soldiers used them with limited success in small skirmishes. About 30 riot-control agents have been developed and used, but their use decreased following the advent of more potent compounds.

After World War I, military and law enforcement agencies used CN (chloroacetophenone) for various purposes until CS (tear gas), a more potent and less toxic compound, synthesized by Corson and Stoughton (hence the nomenclature) in 1928, replaced it in about 1959. The United States used CS extensively in Vietnam primarily for tunnel clearance. The military forces of most countries use CS in training as a confidence builder for the protective mask (the gas chamber exercise), and police forces of many countries (eg,, Ireland, France, Russia, and the US) use it for crowd control or during riots.

Today CN is in commercially available devices for self-protection (Mace, Mace Security International, Inc, Cleveland, OH), but CS and oleoresin capsicum (OC) are fast becoming the favorites among law enforcement agencies. Capsaicin is the active ingredient in OC, commercially called pepper spray. Derived from the resin of cayenne peppers, capsaicin has been used in various ways. In small amounts it is used for pain relief; in larger amounts it is used as an irritant and as a tool of torture. Introduced in 1974 in the United States, it is quickly replacing other riot-control agents used in law enforcement across the country because of its safety and the fact that it can be dispensed as a liquid, foam, or aerosol, or as a powder in paint ball delivery systems. It is best used for individual protection. The United States excludes riot-control agents from international treaty provisions; they may be used in military situations by presidential order, and OC can be used by military law enforcement.

Other riot-control agents include CA (bromobenzyl cyanide), no longer used in the United States because of its low safety margin and caustic nature (it will not be discussed here); CR (dibenz(*b,f*)(1,4)oxazepine), a British agent similar to CS; and DM (also called adamsite), an irritant and vomiting agent. While OC, CS, and CN continue to be used in the United States, CA, CR, and DM are not, but may be used by other nations for riot control.

Physiochemical Characteristics

Unlike most chemical agents, which are liquids under temperate conditions, the riot-control agents CS, CN, CR, and DM are crystallized solids with low vapor pressures and are dispersed as fine particles or in solution. Dispersion devices include small, handheld spray cans; large spray tanks; grenades; and larger weapons. OC is an oily resin, which can be dried to form an off-white powder and aerosolized or combined with a medium such as alcohol or oil to make a liquid or foam spray.

Mechanism of Toxicity

The mechanism of biological activity is less well characterized for riot-control agents than for most other agents. Fortunately, a detailed knowledge of the mechanism of action is not necessary for appropriate medical management. CS and CN are SN_2 alkylating agents (mustard, in contrast, is an SN_1 alkylator) and react readily at nucleophilic sites. Prime targets include sulfhydryl-containing enzymes such as lactic dehydrogenase. In particular, CS reacts rapidly with the disulfhydryl form of lipoic acid, a coenzyme in the pyruvate decarboxylase system. It has been suggested that tissue injury may be related to inactivation of certain of these enzyme systems. Pain can occur without tissue injury and may be bradykinin mediated. CS causes bradykinin release in vivo and in vitro, and elimination of bradykininogen in vivo abolishes the systemic response to CS.

The initial response to aerosolized CS is an increase in blood pressure and irregular respiration, suggestive of the Sherrington pseudoaffective response. Bypassing the pain receptors of the nose and upper airway by endotracheal administration of CS leads to the same decrease in blood pressure; intravenous (IV) injection also causes decreased respiration. These effects suggest that the initial pressor effect and irregular respiration are responses to a noxious stimulus rather than pharmacological effects of CS.

OC produces a burning and painful sensation as it binds to ion-channel receptors in the nervous system, resulting in rapid cell depolarization and a massive release of substance P, a neuropeptide that is a neurotransmitter of pain. This release of high levels of substance P signals the brain that the body is experiencing extreme pain and burning, which continues until the substance P is used up. The body then releases endorphins to inhibit the pain sensation, which can create a period of euphoria (similar to a "runners high") as an after-effect. Those who regularly eat hot peppers are less susceptible to the painful effects of pepper spray. The use of capsaicin in pain-relieving ointments causes a slower release and depletion of substance P, creating an analgesic effect without causing the extreme pain sensation experienced with OC exposure.

Clinical Effects

The main effects of riot-control agents are pain, burning, and irritation of exposed mucous membranes and skin. These effects do not differ appreciably from one agent to another, except in the case of DM, which will be discussed in a separate section.

Eyes

The eye is the organ most sensitive to riot-control agents. Contact with any of the riot-control agents produces a sensation of conjunctival and corneal burning and leads to tearing, blepharospasm, and conjunctival injection. The severe blepharospasm causes the lids to close tightly and produces transient "blindness," an effect that can inhibit the recipient's ability to fight or resist. However, if recipients are able to open their eyes, the vision is near normal even if a significant concentration of the agent persists.

Because these compounds are solids, with the exception of OC, it is possible for a particle or clump to become embedded in the cornea or conjunctiva and cause tissue damage. With the caveat noted below, there is no evidence that this complication has ever occurred; however, those seeking medical care for eye pain after exposure should have their eyes thoroughly decontaminated and undergo thorough ophthalmic examination. It may be necessary to pick out the particles of agent from tissue. The carriers' solvents in some OC sprays can cause corneal erosion, so eyes should be decontaminated with copious amounts of water or baby shampoo and water. Follow-up with an ophthalmologist is indicated if complications appear.

Nose and Mouth

Contact with the delicate mucous membranes of the nose produces a burning sensation, rhinorrhea, and sneezing; a similar burning sensation accompanied by increased salivation occurs after contact with the mouth.

Airways

Inhalation causes burning and irritation of the airways, with bronchorrhea, coughing, and a perception of a "tight" chest or an inability to breathe. In research studies, pulmonary function exams done immediately after exposure have shown minimal alterations. In one reported instance, nine Marines without respiratory protection were exposed to high CS concentrations during training and developed transient pulmonary syndrome. All had coughs and shortness of breath, five had hemoptysis, and four, who needed to be hospitalized, had hypoxia. It was discovered that those hospitalized underwent strenuous physical exercise within 36 to 84 hours after exposure. One week after exposure all nine had normal lung function measured by spirometry before and after exercise.

An inhaled irritating compound might be expected to exacerbate a chronic pulmonary disease such as asthma, emphysema, or bronchitis, but this appears not to happen with CS or CN. The medical care provider should nevertheless anticipate airway problems in individuals with lung disease, particularly if they are exposed to higher than the average field use concentrations. The onset of extreme pain for those exposed to OC has resulted in a few cases of laryngospasm as a reaction to pain. These cases have responded well with standard airway management.

There is no evidence that CS causes permanent lung damage after one or several exposures to field concentrations. Following inhalation of lethal amounts, animals died from severe airway damage 12 to 24 hours postexposure, but survivors from large exposures had minimal or no pulmonary abnormalities. After multiple (50 or more) daily exposures to smaller amounts, animals developed laryngitis and tracheitis.

Skin

Riot-control agents in contact with the skin cause a tingling or burning sensation and may cause erythema, particularly if the skin is raw or freshly abraded (eg, shortly after shaving). The erythema begins several minutes after exposure and generally subsides 45 to 60 minutes after termination of exposure.

Under conditions of high temperature, high humidity, and high concentration of agents such as CS, there may be more severe dermatitis, starting with erythema hours after exposure and followed by vesication. Generally these are second-degree burns similar to sunburn but more severe. Firefighters who entered buildings contaminated with CS after summer riots several decades ago developed these lesions. After stirring up the contaminating particles, they later developed erythema and blisters on their exposed skin. Hypersensitivity may develop for those who have reacted to CS in the past. In one instance, an individual developed generalized vesication and high fever after an uneventful exposure to CS more than 20 years after his only and equally uneventful previous exposure. OC causes skin redness and irritation and possibly, with prolonged exposure to high concentrations, a rash, but not the blistering seen with CS or CN.

Gastrointestinal Tract

Gastrointestinal effects usually do not occur with most riot-control agents (DM is an exception), although there may be retching or vomiting if the agent concentration is high, exposure is prolonged, or the individual is sensitive.

Cardiovascular

A transient increase in heart rate and blood pressure has occurred in people when exposure to riot-control agents was imminent or immediately after exposure. The heart rate and blood pressure returned essentially to pre-test ranges while exposure continued, and may have been caused by the anxiety or the initial pain rather than a pharmacological effect of these agents. This "alarm reaction" may cause adverse effects in those with preexisting cardiovascular disease.

Oral Ingestion

Taking large amounts of capsicum orally can increase the production of stomach acid, but this effect would not be caused by ingestion of minute amounts of OC from a spray or foam. Children occasionally eat CS, and several adults have swallowed CS pellets. Aside from bouts of diarrhea and abdominal cramps (which might have been from the cathartics and antacids used as therapy), their courses have been uneventful. In humans, the median lethal dose (LD_{50}) for CS is an amount unlikely to be ingested, even deliberately. A few animals fed lethal amounts (or greater) of CS had gastric irritation or erosions, and several had signs of intestinal perforation. Recommended therapy after ingestion consists of cathartics, antacids, and surgical observation.

Lethality

Riot-control agents should not be considered nonlethal. They can be lethal when the exposure involves a high concentration or longer period of time. CN, occasionally in combination with DM, has caused deaths in people in a confined space. The confined space contributed to a higher concentration and a longer exposure to the agent. Death generally occurred hours after initial exposure, and postmortem findings were those of severe airway damage. Deaths directly attributed to OC exposure are not easily found in the literature, though theoretically severe laryngospasm could cause respiratory restriction and possible obstruction, hypoxia, and unconsciousness. Those in police custody who died after exposure to OC died from preexisting cardiopulmonary conditions, drug intoxication, or positioning while restrained that restricted breathing, but no deaths have been directly attributed to the actions of OC.

Metabolism

Subjects given lethal amounts of CS by IV or intraperitoneal (IP) administration developed increased blood thiocyanate concentrations hours later, indicating that the malononitrile portion of CS had been metabolized to cyanide. Cyanide was not a factor in causing death (lung damage was). A significant increase in blood concentration of thiocyanate has not been noted after aerosol administration of CS. Several popular databases mention this cyanogenic potential of CS and suggest that treatment of a CS casualty might require therapy for cyanide poisoning (this recommendation is apparently based on the IV or IP administration data). After receiving lethal amounts of CS by inhalation, animals died 12 to 24 hours later from severe airway damage; cyanide was not implicated in their deaths.

OC will cause depletion of substance P over time; once substance P is depleted, pain stops. The body rebuilds substance P stores over several hours to days. OC is absorbed in the body. Those who are exposed to capsaicin for long periods of time, such as in food or topical salves for pain management, have depleted stores of substance P and may not demonstrate as extreme a pain reaction to the administration of OC as others.

DM

DM typically appears as a canary yellow, crystalline solid and has the same unique color when dispensed as a cloud. The effects of usual field concentrations of DM are similar to those of the other riot-control agents, except that DM has little irritancy to the skin. However, at higher concentrations, DM causes nausea, vomiting, and a feeling of generalized malaise. For this reason, it is called a vomiting agent.

Time Course of Effects

Except for those produced by DM, the biological effects from these agents begin seconds after exposure and continue for 15 minutes or so after those exposed exit the contamination to fresh, clean air. The effects from DM begin 2 to 4 minutes after the onset of exposure and may last an hour or two. (This is advantageous militarily, because an individual unaware of the agent will continue to inhale it for several minutes and absorb a larger dose. He or she may then vomit, requiring mask removal, which leads to continued inhalation of agent.)

Differential Diagnosis

Usually the circumstances of exposure help make the diagnosis. The patient history and the physical signs clarify the diagnosis. A patient with conjunctival injection (red eye) and tearing may have a wide differential. Closer examination may reveal normal pupils, whereas a nerve agent exposure would present with constricted pupils. On a battlefield, the sudden onset of burning pain and irritation might lead one to consider lewisite or phosgene oxime exposure, but the signs and symptoms of riot-control agents gradually recede, whereas those from the vesicants worsen.

Laboratory Findings

There are no specific laboratory tests that will confirm the diagnosis. Complications such as infection of a skin lesion will produce the laboratory findings characteristic of the complication.

Medical Management

The effects of exposure to these agents under the usual field conditions generally are self-limiting and require no specific therapy. Most will disappear in 15 to 30 minutes, although erythema may persist for an hour or longer. The following section discusses potential complications occurring only under exceptional circumstances, such as exposure to a very large amount of agent (as in an enclosed space), exposure in adverse weather, or experimental studies in humans or animals. These conditions are not to be expected with normal use of these agents. Less than 1% of exposed people will have effects severe or prolonged enough to cause them to seek medical care. Those who do probably will have eye, airway, or skin complaints. Because there is no antidote for these agents, treatment consists of symptomatic management.

Eyes

The eye should be carefully flushed with water or saline, and impacted particles should be sought. General care consists of a topical solution (many are available) to relieve the irritation and topical antibiotics. An ophthalmologist should be consulted for further evaluation and care. With exposure to OC, milk, vegetable oil, or baby shampoo and copious amounts of water can be effective for eye washing.

Pulmonary

These agents may exacerbate chronic disease or unmask latent disease, although there is little evidence of this. Bronchospasm with wheezing and mild distress continuing hours after exposure may occur in a latent asthmatic. More severe effects and respiratory distress may occur in those with chronic bronchitis or emphysema. Management includes oxygen administration (with assisted ventilation, if necessary), bronchodilators if bronchospasm is present, and specific antibiotics dictated by the results of sputum studies (Gram stains of smears followed by culture). A specialist skilled in the treatment of inhalation injury should be consulted early. Animal studies and very limited human data indicate that maximal effects occur 12 hours after exposure.

Skin

Those with early erythema require reassurance, but no specific therapy unless the condition is severe and prolonged more than an hour or two. Later onset erythema precipitated by a larger exposure in a hot and humid atmosphere is usually more severe and less likely to resolve quickly. It may require the use of soothing compounds such as calamine, camphor, and mentholated creams. Small vesicles should be left intact, but larger ones will ultimately break and should be drained. Irrigation of denuded areas several times a day should be followed by the application of a topical antibiotic. Large, oozing areas have responded to compresses containing substances such as colloidal oatmeal, Burow solution, and other dermatologic preparations.

Decontamination

The crystallized solids CS, CN, CR, and DM can be released from hair, skin, and clothing by flapping the arms or using fans. Although many of these agents are not directly soluble in water, washing with soap and water will effectively remove them from the skin. Washing with soap and water is particularly important for those exposed to the agents for long periods of time, such as an individual operating in a mask confidence chamber. Water increases the pain of OC, so if it is used it should be with copious volumes to help remove the OC from the skin surface. A mild soap, such as baby shampoo, will help loosen resin, as will vegetable oil or alcohol. Casein in milk helps reduce the further release of substance P. Milk, with its lipophilic casein, will also effectively combine with the capsaicin resin to help wash it away.

Triage

A person exposed to the usual field concentrations of riot-control agents will probably not be seen at a triage area. Those presenting with complications should be triaged according to the nature of their injuries.

Return to Duty

Because the effects of field concentrations clear within minutes, the casualty can be returned to duty as soon as possible. Casualties with complications may require evacuation and further medical treatment.

Chapter 7

DECONTAMINATION

Overview

Decontamination is the reduction or removal of hazardous agents. Decontamination of chemical agents may be accomplished by removal of the agents by physical means or by chemical neutralization or detoxification. Patient decontamination is personnel, time, and equipment intensive. Personnel and equipment requirements, although also important, are discussed in other publications and will not be included here. Please refer to USAMRICD's *Field Management of Chemical Casualties Handbook* (the "gold book"; 4th ed, 2014). There are three levels of patient decontamination:

1. **Immediate decontamination.** Primarily performed to protect the individual. Here the contaminated person removes contamination from his or her individual protective equipment (IPE), other equipment, and the skin as quickly as possible after exposure. If the casualty is unable to self-decontaminate, another individual (buddy) provides immediate decontamination.
2. **Patient operational decontamination.** Performed to protect operators of transport vehicles. Unit members remove as much contamination as possible from the casualty's IPE, equipment, and skin, without removing the IPE. This is done to prepare the individual for transport on designated "dirty" evacuation assets to the next level of medical care.
3. **Patient thorough decontamination.** Operators of the patient decontamination station perform this level of decontamination to protect medical facility staff and equipment and to reduce patient contamination. It involves removal of contaminated IPE and a thorough decontamination of any contaminated

skin before the patient enters a medical treatment facility (MTF). The decontamination area should be located about 50 meters downwind from the treatment area (ie, the wind must be blowing from the clean treatment area to the dirty decontamination area).

Prompt removal of an agent from the skin by any nontoxic means is the key to patient decontamination. Immediate decontamination by the soldier can mean the difference between minor and significant medical effects from agent exposure.

The Decontamination Process

Decontamination is the process of removing or reducing a hazardous agent, whether chemical, biological, or radiological, from a person or object. Chemical contamination can present as a vapor, aerosol, liquid, or dry solid. The key reference for patient decontamination in the military is US Army Field Manual 4-02.7, *Health Service Support in a Nuclear, Biological, or Chemical Environment*.

Decontamination is not as critical for those contaminated only by vapor exposure, because vapor will continue to volatilize in the open air; rapidly brushing the hair if vapor is trapped in it and removing a patient's clothing where vapors can be trapped will usually remove the vapor hazard. Exposures to aerosols, liquid, and dry solids will require more thorough decontamination if a patient is to enter a facility where staff are not in protective clothing.

The most important level of decontamination to minimize injury to the patient is immediate decontamination, because it reduces the patient's exposure to a toxic agent. It is most effective if performed within 1 or 2 minutes after exposure, particularly with HD, but the dose will still be reduced to some degree if decontamination is performed later. The goal is to remove the agent from the skin with whatever means are available that are not toxic or abrasive to the skin.

Decontamination studies have been conducted using common household products for the purpose of identifying decontaminants for civilians as well as field expedients for soldiers. Timely use of water, soap and water, or flour, followed by wet tissue wipes, produced results equal, nearly equal, and in some instances better than those produced by the use of Fuller's earth, Dutch powder, and other compounds. (Fuller's earth and Dutch powder are decontamination agents currently fielded by some European countries.) These results were expected because (1) no topical decontaminant has ever shown efficacy with penetrated agent, (2) agents in large enough quantity, especially vesicants, may begin penetrating the skin before complete reactive decontamination (detoxification) takes place, and (3) early physical removal is the most important part of decontamination.

Copious amounts of water or soap and water are effective for washing away most agents. A high volume of water under low pressure should be used, combined with wiping the skin. Fat-based soaps should be used rather than detergents. The fat-based soaps, such as castile soap or other mild liquid soaps, help to emulsify thickened agents such as VX and HD.

Physical removal is imperative because *none* of the chemical means of destroying these agents do so instantaneously. While decontamination preparations such as fresh hypochlorite react rapidly with some agents (eg, the half time for destruction of VX by hypochlorite at a pH of 10 is 1.5 minutes), the half times of destruction for other agents, such as mustard, are much longer. If a large amount of agent is present initially, a longer time is needed to completely neutralize the agent to a harmless substance.

Methods

Three methods of skin decontamination are preferred in the military:

1. Reactive Skin Decontamination Lotion (RSDL) is a new decontaminant that replaced M291 skin decontamination kit. RSDL is a packaged sponge containing a liquid solution that effectively wipes away chemical agents and simultaneously provides oxime protection against nerve agents. It is used on intact skin, but not in open wounds or eyes. RSDL is small and easily carried by service members, making it well suited for field use. Decontamination of the casualty using RSDL does

not eliminate the need for decontamination at a field facility.

2. Soap and water is a low-cost decontaminant that removes agents by washing them off the skin. It is effective for removing chemical, biological, and radiological contaminants. It does not destroy biological agents or neutralize radioactive particles. Both fresh water and sea water have the capacity to remove chemical agents not only through mechanical force but also via slow hydrolysis; however, the generally low solubility and slow rate of diffusion of chemical warfare agents in water significantly limit the hydrolysis rate. The predominant effect of water and water/soap solutions is the physical removal or dilution of agents, although slow hydrolysis does occur, particularly with alkaline soaps. Fat-based liquid soaps (eg, baby shampoo, castile liquid soap, or soft soap) attract and help emulsify chemical agent so that the action of the water can wash it away. Detergents that can dry the skin should not be used. Clean water can be used to irrigate wounds; only copious amounts of water, normal saline, or eye solutions are recommended for the eye.
3. A 0.5% hypochlorite solution with an alkaline pH is an alternate skin decontaminant that can be used when the others are not available and water is limited. It is a solution of nine parts water to one part bleach (which at this dilution is not harmful to the skin). The solution is wiped on the skin and can be rinsed off several minutes later with fresh water. The solution causes a chemical decontamination reaction involving very slow oxidative chlorination and hydrolysis. The term "oxidative chlorination" covers active chlorine chemicals such as hypochlorite. Hypochlorite solutions act universally against the organophosphorus and mustard agents. Both VX and HD contain sulfur atoms that are readily subject to oxidation and hydrolysis. The decontamination effectiveness of these solutions increases as the hypochlorite pH levels go above 8, but these levels are harmful to the skin. Therefore, at the dilution level of 0.5%, the oxidation and hydrolysis effects are present but very limited. Hypochlorite should not be used in abdominal wounds or open chest wounds, on nervous tissue, or in the eye. Irrigation of the abdomen may lead to adhesions and is therefore also contraindicated. The use of hypochlorite

in the thoracic cavity may be less of a problem, but the hazard is still unknown.

Certification of Decontamination

Certification of decontamination for chemical agents is accomplished by any of the following: processing through the decontamination station, M8 paper, the Joint Chemical Agent Detector (JCAD), or the Improved Chemical Agent Monitor (ICAM). If proper procedure is followed, the possibility of admitting a contaminated casualty to an MTF is extremely small.

Wound Decontamination

The initial management of a casualty contaminated by chemical agents requires removal of IPE and skin decontamination before treatment at an MTF. When thorough decontamination is performed, contaminated bandages are removed and wounds are flushed with sterile water. Any contaminated debris (such as clothing in the wound that may hold agent) is irrigated and removed from the wound by decontaminated gloved hands, instruments, or another no-touch technique. The bandages are then replaced only if bleeding recurs or the wound needs protection from further contamination. Contaminated tourniquets are replaced with clean tourniquets and the sites of the original tourniquets decontaminated. Splints are thoroughly decontaminated by rinsing with a 0.5% hypochlorite solution or copious amounts of soap and water, but should only be removed by a physician or a medic directly supervised by a physician.

General Considerations

Of the agents discussed, only two types, vesicants and nerve agents, may present a hazard from wound contamination. Cyanide is quite volatile, so it is extremely unlikely that liquid cyanide will remain in a wound, and it requires a very large amount of liquid cyanide to produce vapor adequate to cause effects.

Mustard converts to a cyclic compound within minutes of absorption into a biological milieu, and the compound rapidly (within minutes) reacts with components of the wound: blood, necrotic tissue, and the remaining viable tissue. If the amount of bleeding and tissue damage is small, mustard rapidly enters the surrounding viable tissue, where it will quickly biotransform and attach to tissue components. Its biological behavior will be much like an intramuscular absorption of the agent.

Although nerve agents cause toxic effects by their very rapid attachment to the enzyme acetylcholinesterase, they also quickly react with other enzymes and tissue components. As with mustard, the blood and necrotic tissue of the wound will buffer nerve agents. Nerve agent that reaches viable tissue will be rapidly absorbed, and since the toxicity of nerve agents is quite high (a lethal amount is a small drop), it is unlikely that casualties who have had much nerve agent in a wound will survive to reach medical care. Potential risk to the surgeon from possibly contaminated wounds arises from agent on foreign bodies in the wound and from thickened agents.

Thickened Agent

Thickened agents are chemical agents that have been mixed with another substance (commonly an acrylate) to increase their persistency. They do not dissolve as quickly in biological fluids, nor are they absorbed by tissue as rapidly as other agents. Similarly, VX, although not a thickened agent, is absorbed less quickly and may persist in the wound longer than other nerve agents.

Casualties with thickened nerve agents in wounds are unlikely to survive. Thickened HD has delayed systemic toxicity and can persist in wounds even when any large fragments of cloth have been removed. Though the vapor hazard to surgical personnel is extremely low, contact hazard from thickened agents does remain and precautions should always be taken.

No country is currently known to stockpile thickened agents. In a chemical attack, the intelligence and chemical staffs should be able to identify thickened agents and alert medical personnel of their use.

Off-Gassing

The risk from vapor off-gassing from chemically contaminated shrapnel and cloth in wounds is very low and not significant.

Furthermore, there is no vapor release from contaminated wounds without foreign bodies. Off-gassing from a wound during surgical exploration will be negligible (or zero). No eye injury will result from off-gassing from any of the agents. A chemical-protective mask is not required for surgical personnel.

Foreign Material

The contamination of wounds with mustard or nerve agents is largely confined to the foreign material (eg, uniform and protective garment in the wound). The removal of this cloth from the wound effectively eliminates the hazard. There is little chemical risk associated with individual fibers left in the wound. No further decontamination of the wound for chemical agent is necessary.

Wound Exploration and Debridement

During exploration and debridement, surgeons and their assistants are advised to wear a pair of well-fitting (thin), butyl rubber gloves or double latex surgical gloves and to change them often until they are certain there are no foreign bodies or thickened agents in the wound. This is especially important where puncture is likely because of the presence of bone spicules or metal fragments.

The wound should be explored with surgical instruments rather than with fingers. Pieces of cloth and associated debris must be quickly disposed of in a container of 5% hypochlorite. The wound can then be checked with the ICAM, which may direct the surgeon to further retained material. It takes about 30 seconds to get a stable reading from the ICAM; a rapid pass over the wound will not detect remaining contamination. The wound is debrided and excised according to the usual procedures, maintaining a no-touch technique. Removed fragments of tissue are placed into hypochlorite. Tissue such as an amputated limbs should be placed in a sealable, chemical-proof plastic or rubber bag.

Hypochlorite solution (0.5%) may be instilled into noncavity wounds following the removal of contaminated cloth. This solution should be removed by suction. Within 5 minutes, this contaminated solution will be neutralized and nonhazardous. Subsequent irrigation with saline or other surgical solutions should be performed.

Surgical practices should be effective for the majority of wounds in identifying and removing the focus of remaining agent within the peritoneum. Saline, hydrogen peroxide, or other irrigating solutions may not decontaminate agents, but may dislodge material for recovery by aspiration. The irrigation solution should not be swabbed out manually with surgical sponges. The risk to patients and medical attendants is minuscule; however, safe practice suggests that any irrigation solution should be considered potentially contaminated. Following aspiration by suction, the suction apparatus and the solution should be disposed of in a solution of 5% hypochlorite.

Superficial wounds should be thoroughly wiped with soap and water or a 0.5% hypochlorite solution and subsequent irrigation with normal saline.

Instruments that have become contaminated should be placed in 5% hypochlorite for 10 minutes prior to normal cleansing and sterilization. Reusable linen should be checked with the ICAM or M8 paper for contamination; if found to be contaminated, it should be disposed of in a 5% to 10% hypochlorite solution.

Conclusion

Decontamination at the MTF is directed toward (1) eliminating agent transfer to the patient during removal of protective clothing, (2) decontaminating or containing contaminated clothing and personal equipment, and (3) maintaining an uncontaminated MTF. Current doctrine specifies the use of RSDL, soap and water, or a 0.5% hypochlorite solution. These decontaminants have been tested and found to be effective when used appropriately.

Chapter 8

CASUALTY MANAGEMENT IN A CONTAMINATED AREA

Overview

In a contaminated environment, casualties enter a medical treatment facility (MTF) through the patient decontamination site (PDS). This occurs at all levels of medical care where contaminated casualties might be received. The purpose of the PDS is to remove all contamination, or as much as possible, from the casualty before he or she enters the clean MTF; this ensures that unprotected medical staff inside the facility are not made ill or become cross-contaminated by agent on the arriving patient. The key military reference for the decontamination of patients is US Army Field Manual 4-02.7, *Health Service Support in a Nuclear, Biological, or Chemical Environment,* which provides detailed instructions on establishing and operating a PDS. The key reference for the establishment of stateside MTF patient decontamination is the Occupational Safety and Health (OSHA) *Best Practices for Hospital-Based First Receivers of Victims from Mass Casualty Incidents Involving the Release of Hazardous Substances* (January 2005). This section outlines the key points found in those documents. PDS diagrams are also found in Appendix A.

Zones of Contamination

Zones of contamination (hot, warm, and cold) are established at both the incident or attack location and the PDS. The zones at each location are entirely separate. All casualties arriving at a PDS should be presumed contaminated until confirmed otherwise.

- **Hot Zone.** The area directly contaminated by chemical, biological, radiological, or nuclear agents. In combat, it is the contaminated battlefield or toxic industrial material release site (eg, factory storage tank or terrorist bomb). Casualties usually undergo immediate decontamination in the hot zone or on the periphery of it.

- **Warm Zone**. An area where low levels of dry, liquid, and vapor contamination can be expected once contaminated individuals enter. The contamination hazard is essentially the agent that remains on patients brought into this area. In this zone immediate, patient operational, and patient thorough decontamination take place. The PDS is initially set up in an area free of contamination, which becomes part of the warm zone once contaminated casualties begin to arrive.
- **Cold Zone**. An area free from liquid, dry, and vapor contamination. All personnel and patients entering this zone have been decontaminated. Protective ensemble and mask are usually not required for personnel in the cold zone unless the area becomes contaminated. Standard precautions must be practiced if a patient is infectious with a biological agent.

In some contexts the PDS terms "warm" and "hot" can be used synonymously with "dirty," and the term "cold" be used interchangeably with the term "clean."

The principal components of the PDS are:

- entry control point and arrival point
- triage area
- emergency treatment area
- decontamination areas
- "hot line"(separating the contaminated from the clean areas)

After crossing the hot line, the casualty enters the clean triage and treatment area. From there, the now contamination-free casualty is brought into the MTF or prepared for "clean" disposition to another MTF. The size of the MTF will dictate the personnel support needed to staff a functional PDS. At a battalion aid station, for example, staffing is limited and the same senior medical noncommissioned officer serving as the triage officer may also provide emergency care. The decontamination areas will be staffed by a limited number of augmented personnel, and very limited medical care can be provided in the clean treatment area. At larger MTFs a medical professional will be available to perform triage and others to provide emergency care. There will be more decontamination lanes and more augmentees to staff them. If augmented personnel are not plentiful, the decontamination team can be supplemented by nonmedical personnel from the hospital staff. Staffing a PDS can take 8 to 39 people, depending on its size and the time it needs to remain in operation. The following is intended as an introduction to each of these stations. More detailed information can be found in USAMRICD's *Field Management of Chemical Casualties Handbook* (the "gold book"; 4th ed, 2014) or the references noted previously.

Key Components of a Patient Decontamination Site

All PDS operations must have the following key components to operate effectively.

Dirty Side

Protection. All staff on this side of the PDS wear MOPP (mission-oriented protective posture) level IV or OSHA personal protective equipment level C.

Entry control point and arrival area. Patients pass through the entry control point, where access to the PDS is controlled. Vehicles with casualties then proceed to the arrival point, where they are unloaded. This area is staffed by augmentees. Key activities here are (1) routing of vehicles, (2) unloading of vehicles, and (3) quick pat down searches to remove ordinance from patients. All staff are in MOPP level IV when contaminated patients arrive.

Warm side triage area. The triage area is located near the arrival area; patients are moved here from the arrival point. Here casualties are simultaneously triaged according to their need for medical care, their priority for patient thorough decontamination, and their priority for evacuation to the next role of care. Within the triage area casualties are moved to either the immediate (warm side emergency medical treatment [EMT] area), delayed, minimal, or expectant treatment areas. Patients are retriaged as they progress through the EMT and decontamination and as their condition changes. The following placement of treatment areas in relation to the decontamination lanes is suggested to improve patient flow through the PDS.

- *Immediate* patients are moved to the warm side EMT area. This area is located between patient triage (closer to triage to minimize the time it takes to move from triage to dirty EMT) and the entrance to the litter decontamination lanes. This way a patient can be moved to litter decontamination without interfering with the traffic flow from other patient groups.
- The *delayed* patient area should be positioned nearer to the entrance to both the litter and ambulatory decontamination lines. This way delayed patients can be processed through either the litter or ambulatory lanes as they become available.
- *Minimal* patients should be positioned near the ambulatory patient area so that if medical care on the clean side of the hot line is needed, they can be processed through the ambulatory lane when it becomes available without interfering with the flow to the litter lanes.
- *Expectant* patients should be located near the EMT area, but farther away from the decontamination lanes so they can be retriaged and stabilized for decontamination if the EMT area no longer has patients in it.

Warm side EMT area. Patients triaged as immediate for medical treatment are sent to this area until their condition is stabilized for patient thorough decontamination or for dirty evacuation to another medical facility. An initial quantity of medical supplies is located in this area to provide antidotes to chemical agents, bandages for wounds, equipment to establish intravenous (IV) access, intubation equipment to establish emergency airways, and decontamination kits to provide immediate or operational decontamination to patients. It is important to place only enough supplies here for the anticipated number of patients so that unused supplies are not in danger of contamination. The warm side EMT area should be large enough to expand and handle an influx of patients. Staffing should consist of trained and experienced medics (eg, emergency medical technicians, corpsmen), nurses, or physician assistants.

Warm side disposition (dirty evacuation). Located in the vicinity of the warm side EMT, here patients remain in protective ensemble and undergo operational decontamination and staging for dirty evacuation (by ground, water, or rotor-wing aircraft) to another MTF where adequate resources are available to care for them.

Contaminated waste dump. This area is located at least 75 m downwind from the hot line. Bags of contaminated clothing and bandages are taken to the dump, where they are buried and marked with appropriate hazard markers. The position is communicated to headquarters so that the waste can be disposed of properly.

Temporary morgue. A shaded area located on the warm side is set up where the contaminated remains of those who die while being processed through the PDS are stored. These remains stay on the warm side of the hot line and are handled in accordance with theater policy until they are retrieved by the services unit that turns them over to mortuary affairs.

Litter patient decontamination lane. Located between the warm side EMT and the hot line, this area is where litter patients have their clothing removed, contaminated bandages and splints replaced, and personal effects and field medical card (FMC) placed in plastic, zip-lock bags, and where they are decontaminated. Patients must be medically stable enough to undergo decontamination before they are brought to this area. Those performing decontamination also wear a toxicological agent protective (TAP) apron over their protective ensemble to keep the ensemble dry and allow the aprons to be decontaminated before conducting patient transfers. With the exception of the Air Force and some Navy units who have trained medical teams throughout the decontamination process, this area is staffed by augmentees who are closely supervised by an medic.

Ambulatory patient decontamination lane. This area is usually located parallel to the litter patient decontamination lane. Ambulatory patients who need to see the physicians at the MTF are processed through this area, where they have their clothing removed, contaminated bandages and splints replaced, and personal effects and FMC placed in plastic, zip-lock bags, and where they are decontaminated. Ambulatory individuals without medical complaints requiring care at the MTF are treated in the treatment area and returned to their unit without undergoing decontamination or crossing the hot line, or they are processed through troop decontamination lanes and not through the medical ambulatory decontamination lane. Those performing decontamination also wear a TAP apron to keep their protective ensemble dry. This area is usually manned by at least one medic, and other augmentees if available, to supervise ambulatory patients as they are processed through the line and assist one another.

Contamination check area. This area is located between the decontamination lanes and the hot line. Here, completeness of decontamination is checked using the appropriate monitoring devices (eg, Improved Chemical Agent Monitor [ICAM] or M8 paper). Zip-lock bags containing the patient's personal items can also be unzipped and the monitors used to check for contamination of the items inside. The decontamination check of patients may not be necessary where fully plumbed decontamination tents provide adequate soap and water for a thorough wash.

Litter decontamination station. Here, warm side litters are washed and readied for reuse. Buckets and sponges with 5% hypochlorite solution are available as well as water to rinse litters. With a shower/roller system, litters need only to be sent back through the decontamination station for a wash with soap and water.

Weapons and contaminated personal effects storage area. Here, patient weapons and personal effects are secured and inventoried. Items from this area are decontaminated and moved through the contamination check area before being sent across the hot line. If personnel are limited, this area may need to be well organized and under the observation of personnel serving as security augmentees.

Warm side rest area. A shaded area where the PDS team can rest and drink water while remaining in their protective ensemble.

Hot line and shuffle pit. The hot line separates the PDS warm zone (dirty side) from the cold zone (clean side) where the MTF is located. *No liquid or solid contamination may cross the hot line.* The line must be indicated in some way (eg, by a barrier, tape line, or air lock) so that all personnel know they cannot cross the line until they are properly decontaminated. In the battlefield it is best to indicate this area with a specific barrier, such as concertina wire, to protect the medical facility. Shuffle pits or boot rinses are located at openings along the hot line to ensure that footwear worn by individuals moving across the hot line is decontaminated. At the hot line, information on the patient's FMC is transferred to a clean card, and litter patients are transferred to a clean litter to ensure that no contaminated cards or litters cross the hot line. A blanket is also placed on the patient once they are transferred to a clean litter. Team members on the clean side receive the patient. Staffing on the dirty side consists of the team in TAP aprons who decontaminated the patient and the warm side medic, if available. Receiving members consist of one medic and at least two augmentees for litter patients and one augmentee for ambulatory patients.

Vapor control line. This line is typically upwind of the hot line by approximately 10 meters. Patients and PDS team members remain masked until they cross this line. The line can be established using chemical vapor detectors such as the Automatic Chemical Agent Detection Alarm.

Clean Side

Protection. Personnel assigned to this area do not need to wear protective equipment because the patients in here are free from contamination. When processing infectious biological casualties, staff should practice universal precautions and wear appropriate respiratory protection.

Triage/EMT area (cold zone). Located beyond the hot line and vapor control line, this contamination-free area is where patients are retriaged and treated. It can be a holding and staging area for admission to the MTF, for clean evacuation to another MTF, or for ambulance transport from a co-located (troop and patient) PDS to a nearby MTF.

Disposition/clean evacuation (cold zone). This area is adjacent to the cold zone triage / EMT. From this area, contamination-free patients who have been stabilized are staged for transport to another treatment facility.

Supply point. This point is located outside the vapor control line. PDS supplies are kept here and are handed across the hot line to the warm side when needed.

Patient Decontamination Site Critical Concerns

Warm Side Triage

It is important that the triage officer be practiced enough to effectively triage patients so that the PDS is not overwhelmed with patients who can be treated on the warm side and returned to their unit; who should be "dirty evacuated" to a larger MTF (if possible); or who can be stabilized in the warm area until they are ready for decontamination. The triage officer might be a senior medic in a battalion aid station. In larger medical units the triage officer might be a physician or physician's assistant. The triage officer's ability to evaluate the casualty will be limited because both the officer and the casualty will be in MOPP Level IV.

Warm Side Emergency Medical Care

Those casualties needing immediate care will be sent to the warm side EMT. Casualties classified as minimal might also be sent to this area, if the appropriate care can be provided in a contaminated environment, so that they can be returned to duty quickly and lessen the workload on the decontamination teams. However, the types of injuries that can be treated without breaking the integrity of the protective garment are small (although antidotes may be administered without breaking a garment's seal). Once the garment's integrity is violated, the minimal casualty will need to be treated and sent through troop decontamination to don replacement individual protective equipment (IPE) before being returned to the battle area. Arrangements must be made with supported units to have replacement IPE available for these casualties. Decontaminated litter patients should be placed in a patient protective wrap if they need to be transported on dirty evacuation assets or through contaminated areas.

Casualties classified as delayed will be sent through the PDS for decontamination if they require care in the clean treatment area. Otherwise, they will be dirty evacuated to the next level of care that can better handle them. The expectant casualty will be temporarily set aside, adjacent to the warm side EMT, for later reevaluation when there are no more patients in the EMT station.

The amount of vapor arising from patient IPE should not be enough to preclude an apneic patient from being ventilated. Ideally, in a battlefield environment a resuscitation device, individual chemical (RDIC), with its filtered "ambu-bag" should be used. Ventilation of a newly apneic patient will be limited more by the lack of personnel to squeeze the ambu-bag than by the risk of forcing more chemical vapor into the casualty's lungs. IV injections can be given and fluids started after decontamination of the skin at the IV insertion site and the care provider's gloves. Minor suturing can be done in this area using the same precautions. The time needed by the single medical care provider to perform these procedures is probably the limiting consideration, rather than the risk of further contamination.

Preventing Musculoskeletal and Heat Injury

Patient triage, treatment, and decontamination involve moderate and heavy work. This can create heat injury and increase accident frequency as overheated workers overlook safety procedures. A safety officer must be appointed for operations on the warm side of the PDS. This can be the officer in charge, noncommissioned officer in charge, or some other individual. It must be someone who can observe the PDS workers, travel freely around the PDS, and manage work/rest cycles.

Worker musculoskeletal injury can easily occur from lifting patients, carrying litters, or falling while wearing protective ensemble. To reduce these injuries, clear routes within the PDS to reduce tripping hazards; establish decontamination lanes far apart to reduce clutter; enforce frequent garbage bag removal to reduce trip hazards; train and enforce safe lifting techniques; ensure there are adequate rest breaks; and use work-saving equipment such as NATO litter carriers, if available.

Work/rest cycles (Table 8-1) should be carried out on the warm side of the hot line. Enforcing adequate worker rest helps ensure adequate hydration, gives the body an opportunity to get rid of excessive heat, slows down the production of internal body heat created during physical work, and provides greater blood flow to the skin. Wearing IPE generates heat that is not easily dissipated by the process of sweating because the wearer's skin does not contact the air. Wearing protective overgarments adds 10°F (5.6°C) to the wet bulb globe temperature (WBGT) index, and wearing body armor increases it by another 5°F (2.8°C). The

Table 8-1. Work/Rest Cycles

		Moderate Work		Hard Work	
Heat Category	WBGT Index (°F)	Work/ Rest (Min)	Water Intake Qt/H	Work/ Rest (Min)	Water Intake Qt/H
1 (White)	78–81.9	NL	3/4	40/20	3/4
2 (Green)	82–84.9	50/10	3/4	30/30	1
3 (Yellow)	85–87.9	40/20	3/4	30/30	1
4 (Red)	88–89.9	30/30	3/4	20/40	1
5 (Black)	> 90	20/40	1	10/50	1

NL: not limited (60 minutes work with minimal rest)
WBGT: wet bulb globe temperature

following are common forms of heat injury.

Heat stroke. *Cause:* The body's temperature regulatory system fails and sweating becomes inadequate. *Signs and symptoms:* Body temperature is usually 105°F (40.5°C) or higher. The victim is mentally confused, delirious, perhaps in convulsions, or unconscious. *Medical attention:* First-aid must be administered immediately because death can occur without rapid treatment. Move the victim to a cool shaded area. Process the victim quickly across the hot line. Remove the victim's IPE, soak the underclothing with water, and fan the patient to increase cooling. Evacuate to nearest MTF for monitored fluid replacement.

Heat exhaustion. *Cause*: Loss of large amounts of fluid by sweating, sometimes with excessive loss of salt. *Signs and symptoms:* Sweating, extreme weakness or fatigue; patient may show giddiness, nausea, or headache; symptoms may resemble those of early heat stroke. The skin is clammy and moist, the complexion is pale and flushed, and body temperature is normal or slightly elevated. The victim may lose consciousness. *Medical attention:* Notify medical personnel immediately. Move the victim to a cool place to rest. Process the victim across the hot line as operation tempo permits. Encourage liquid intake and monitor status.

Heat cramps. *Cause:* Painful spasms of the muscles in those who sweat profusely and drink large quantities of water, but do not adequately replace salt loss. *Medical attention:* Cramps may occur during or after work hours and may be relieved by taking salted liquids by mouth. Move the individual to the warm side rest area and seek medical attention. *Return to work:* patient can be put in a less physically demanding position if the condition improves; or process the patient across the hot line when operations tempo allows.

Fainting. *Cause:* Heat causes blood vessels in the skin and lower part of the body to enlarge to try to cool the body. The blood may pool there rather than return to the heart to be pumped to the brain, causing the person to faint. Typically seen in a worker who is unaccustomed to hot environments. *Medical attention:* The worker should lie down in the warm side rest area. Elevate the legs and seek medical advice. Return the individual to duty when recovered or process across the hot line when operation tempo allows.

Underhydration and overhydration. A worker may produce 2 to 3 gallons of sweat in the course of a day's work. Do not depend on thirst to signal when and how much to drink; 5 to 7 ounces of liquid should be consumed every 15 to 20 minutes. However, water intake should not exceed 1 quart per hour or 12 quarts per day. Excessive water consumption can dilute the salt content of the blood to the point where it interferes with brain, heart, and muscle function, which can result in heart attack and seizure.

Chapter 9

INDIVIDUAL PROTECTIVE EQUIPMENT

This overview is divided into four sections: (1) individual protection, (2) individual decontamination, (3) detection and alarms, and (4) patient protective equipment. For further information on these items, see the current technical manual for each piece of equipment.

Individual Protection

This section includes standard "A" individual protective equipment (IPE) issued to each soldier depending on his or her military occupational specialty and consisting of the following items:

- M40A1 Chemical Biological Field Protective Mask
- M42A2 Chemical Biological Combat Vehicle Protective Mask
- M45 Air Crew/Land Warrior Chem-Bio Mask System
- MCU-2A/P Protective Mask
- M50 Field Protective Joint Service General Purpose Mask (JSGPM)
- M51 Combat Vehicle Joint Service General Purpose Mask (JSGPM)
- M53 Chemical-Biological Protective Mask
- Joint Service Lightweight Integrated Suit Technology (JSLIST)
- Chemical/Biological/Radiological/Nuclear Lightweight Overboots Alternative Footwear Solution (AFS)
- JSLIST Joint Block 2 Glove Upgrade (JB2GU)

M40A1, M42A2, and M45 Masks

The M40A1, M42A2, and M45 (serial numbers TM-3-4240-346-10 and TM-3-4240-348-10) are three variations of a protective mask sharing many of the same design characteristics, capabilities, and features. Each mask has been designed for very specific mission requirements, such as aircraft or combat vehicle operation. Technical information on overall mask operations will be covered here.

These protective masks provide users with respiratory, eye, and face protection against chemical and biological agents and radioactive fallout particles. If a mask is properly fitted and worn correctly, it provides a gas-tight face seal, which prevents contaminated air from reaching the wearer's respiratory, ocular, and dermal systems. These masks have not been designed for use in toxic industrial chemical (TIC) environments and are known to be ineffective against chemicals such as ammonia and carbon monoxide. For this reason, personnel exposed to unidentified TICs should consider the masks as escape devices only, and leave the contaminated area as rapidly as possible. The masks are also not suitable for confined spaces where oxygen is insufficient to support life.

Each mask is constructed of silicone rubber with an in-turned sealing surface so that it can form a comfortable seal on the wearer's face, an external second skin for additional protection. A binocular eye lens system is used for improved vision, with clear and tinted "outserts" to provide eye protection against lasers and low speed fragmentation. Optical inserts may be used if the user requires corrective lenses. An elastic head harness secures the mask to the user's face. Other common features include front and side "voicemitters" for face-to-face and phone communications, and each mask is furnished with drinking tubes to allow for hydration.

A key design feature of each of the discussed protective masks is the use of a standard C2A1 NATO threaded filter canister. The canister is externally mounted and may be mounted on the left or right side of the face piece, depending on the preference of the user. The C2A1 canister must be disposed of in accordance with state and local environmental laws.

MCU-2A/P Mask

The MCU-2A / P series mask (Air Force Technical Order 14P4-15-1) is designed to protect the face, eyes, and respiratory tract of the user from tactical concentrations of chemical and biological agents, toxins, and radioactive fallout particles. The mask has a unimolded, silicone rubber face piece and a single flexible lens bonded onto the face piece. The large lens gives the user a wide field of vision. It has a single filter and two voicemitters, one on the front of the mask for speaking directly into a telephone or radio handset and one at the side to allow personnel nearby to hear. A nose cup with two inlet valves fits over the nose and mouth. It directs incoming air across the inside of the lens to reduce fogging. The mask has a drinking tube that connects to a canteen with an M1 cap. The mask is not authorized for use during TIC spills, and the mask is not effective against chemicals such as ammonia, chlorine, or carbon monoxide fumes. The mask is not effective in confined spaces where oxygen levels are insufficient to sustain life.

M50 and M51 Masks

The JSGPM (TM-3-4240-542-13&P) is the first joint service protective mask designed to replace the M40 / M42 series of masks, mask carrier, and accessories for the US Army and Marine Corps ground and combat vehicle operations and the MCU-2 / P series of masks for the Air Force and Navy shore-based and shipboard applications. The JSGPM is provided in two models with individual stock numbers to support major operational modes: the M50 for field use and the M51 for use in combat vehicles.

The M50 and M51 face piece assemblies are built on a butyl and silicone rubber face blank with an inverted peripheral face seal and an integrated chin cup. The face piece assembly forms a comfortable seal on the wearer's face and protects the face, eyes, and respiratory tract from chemical and biological agents, designated TICs, and radiological particulates. The face piece assembly incorporates a flexible, single polyurethane eye lens that provides a widened and uninterupted field of vision compared to the M40 mask. A front module assembly provides a direct speech capability and integrates the exhalation disk valve, drinking system components, and communications interface. Filtration is provided by two filter mount assemblies (left and right) that integrate the air inlet disk valves and self-sealing disk valves, and a nose cup that controls the flow of air throughout the mask and prevents fogging of the eye lens during breathing.

Both masks use twin M61 filters, positioned on either side of the face piece, to provide protection against nuclear, biological, and chemical threats. The filters are attached to the filter mount using a twist and lock mechanism. The M51 uses the combat vehicle hose assembly to connect the mask to the vehicle collective protection system. Additionally, a protective hood is provided for JSLIST type VII users to protect the head and neck from exposure to agents because these suits lack a hood.

M53 Mask

The M53 mask (TM-3-4240-541-12&P) is specially designed to meet US Special Operations requirements; it is not a standard mask issued to other service members. The M53 face piece assembly is built on a butyl and silicone rubber face blank with an inverted peripheral face seal and an integrated chin cup. The face piece assembly forms a comfortable seal on the wearer's face and protects the face, eyes, and respiratory tract from chemical and biological agents, certain TICs, and radiological particulates. The face piece assembly incorporates a single, flexible, polyurethane eye lens; a variable resistance exhalation unit that allows for operations in negative pressure, powered air purifying respirator, self-contained breathing apparatus, and closed circuit breathing apparatus modes; drinking system components; a communications interface; and single filter mount assemblies with a 40-mm NATO thread that integrates the inlet disk valve and air deflector. The mask uses a single general purpose filter, positioned on the side of the face, to provide protection against nuclear, biological, and chemical threats and certain TICs. A particulate filter is also available as an additional authorization list item. A protective hood is provided for JSLIST type VII users.

Joint Service Lightweight Integrated Suit Technology

The JSLIST (TM-10-8415-220-10) consists of a two-piece garment system that provides protection from radiological, biological, toxins, and chemical contaminants. The JSLIST provides multiple improvements over legacy protective garments, including reduced thermal burden, reduced weight, and increased potential wear time. The garment is assembled with a rip-stop outer shell of 50% nylon and 50% cotton poplin, and an interior liner of filter fabric that uses carbon sphere beads to reduce chemical and biological contamination. The garment is manufactured in two distinct designs: type II and type VII. The type II has a hood and is used for most applications; the type VII has a stand-up collar and is used by Special Operations personnel. The JSLIST is currently available in desert camouflage, woodland, and universal camouflage.

The two JSLIST components are a coat and trousers. Each component is separately packaged in a factory sealed vacuum bag containing the ensemble item and a resealable bag. Once the garment has been removed from the vacuum-sealed packaging, it provides 45 days of wear and 120 days of service life. The JSLIST provides up to 24 hours of protection against chemical and biological agents in solid, liquid, or vapor form within the stated maximum wear time. The garment will also protect against alpha and beta radioactive particles. To properly maintain and store the JSLIST when not in use, the garment should be placed in the furnished resealable bag.

The JSLIST ensemble should be worn in all environments under threat of an imminent nuclear, biological, or chemical attack or after chemical operations have been initiated. The garment can be laundered up to six times by field methods; however, once the garment has been contaminated, the soldier must replace it as soon as mission permits by using mission-oriented protective posture (MOPP) gear exchange procedures.

The JSLIST adds weight to the soldier's workload. In addition, the garment reduces heat exchange with the environment and may add, depending on the level of exertion, 10 °F to 15°F to the wearer's ambient temperature and heat burden. When wearing the JSLIST at MOPP 1 or MOPP 2 and complete encapsulation is not required, certain modifications to the uniform are authorized:

- The trouser leg Velcro (Velcro Industries, Manchester, NH) closures may be opened.
- The waist tabs may be loosened.
- The jacket may be unzipped.
- The sleeve Velcro closures may be opened.

This overall loosening of the JSLIST will allow heat to escape because walking and other movements induce a bellows action of the suit against underlying clothing and skin.

Alternative Footwear Solution

The AFS is a chemical-biological protective overboot that is worn over normal combat footwear. It is issued with the JSLIST and available in sizes X-small to XX-large. The AFS will provide 24 hours of protection in a chemical or biological contaminated environment. The overboots can be worn for up to 376 hours over 45 days in an uncontaminated environment. AFS has an antislip ridge tread pattern for improved traction, an antistatic surface, and fully sealed and vulcanized seams, as well as three sets of buttons with a butyl rubber securing strap for each set. The adjustable securing strap is symmetrical and can be released from either side of the overboot. AFS overboots contaminated with petroleum, oil, and lubricants should be wiped off within 2 minutes and air-dried. If contaminants remain more than 2 minutes, the boot protection may be degraded. In such instances, the overboots must be replaced as soon as possible.

Joint Service Lightweight Integrated Suit Technology Block 2 Glove Upgrade

The JB2GU provides 24 hours of chemical and biological protection from battlefield concentrations of all known agents for up to 30 days of wear. The glove provides enhanced tactility, dexterity, durability, and comfort over legacy systems and can be worn in all climates. These qualities satisfy a broader spectrum of ground, shipboard, and aviation requirements. The JB2GU comes in two variants: flame-resistant (FR) and non–flame-resistant (nFR). The FR variant combines a Nomex (DuPont, Wilmington, DE) and leather outer glove with an inner chemical protective liner for aviators and combat vehicle crews. The nFR variant is a molded glove made from compounded butyl rubber and comes with a removable protective liner for sweat management. The nFR glove is primarily for ground forces, and is available in sizes S to XL.

Individual Decontamination

The preceding section provided an overview of the primary US military IPE, which, when used correctly, will prevent contact with chemical agents in typical battlefield concentrations. The problem of decontamination arises when soldiers, because of poor training, poor discipline, or bad luck, become exposed to liquid agent despite the availability of protective masks and clothing.

This section addresses two decontamination kits currently in the US inventory: (1) the Joint Service Personnel/Skin Decontamination System (JSPDS), also known as Reactive Skin Decontamination Lotion (RSDL), and (2) the M295 Individual Equipment Decontamination Kit. Both kits are fairly simple in design and function, and instructions for their use are straightforward and easily committed to memory. Because of the potency of liquid nerve agents and the rapidly occurring tissue damage caused by vesicants, every soldier must be able to conduct an effective decontamination of all exposed skin without referring to the printed instructions.

Joint Service Personnel/Skin Decontamination System

The JSPDS, or RSDL (NSN-6505-01-507-5074; TM-3-6505-001-10), is an individually carried skin decontamination kit approved by the US Food and Drug Administration. RSDL provides the soldier with the ability to decontaminate the skin after exposure to chemical or biological warfare agents, in support of immediate and thorough personnel decontamination operations. The kit consists of decontaminants and applicators required to immediately reduce morbidity and mortality resulting from chemical warfare agent contamination of the skin. The system's applicators are preimpregnated with RSDL, a potassium solution dissolved in a special solvent and water that facilitates the reaction of decontamination between the potassium salt and the chemical agent. The lotion decontaminates the warfare agents mustard (HD), soman (GD), and VX as well as T-2 mycotoxins on skin to a level that eliminates toxic effects better than the previous M291 kit. Each packet will decontaminate an area of 1,300 cm^2. The system can be used in temperatures ranging from -25°F (-32°C) to 130°F (54°C). In addition to immediate decontamination of the user's skin, it can be used to decontaminate individual equipment, weapons, and other casualties (on unbroken skin).

M295 Individual Equipment Decontamination Kit

The M295 (NSN-4230-01-357-8456; TM-3-4230-235-10) is a handheld kit used to apply decontaminant to the individual's personal equipment. Each kit consists of a carrying pouch, which contains four sealed packets, each with a wipe-down mitt containing 22 g of powder (enough to perform two complete individual equipment decontamination operations). Each packet is designed to fit comfortably within a pocket of the JSLIST overgarment trousers. The decontaminating powder in the mitt is contained within a pad material with a polyethylene film backing. In use, powder from the mitt is allowed to flow freely through the pad material. Decontamination is accomplished through sorption of contamination by both the pad and the decontaminating powder. The M295 is issued in boxes of 20. The kits should be stored at the squad level in a box capable of being decontaminated.

Detection and Alarms

This section will describe the equipment issued for detection and identification of chemical agent liquid and vapor in the environment. For both the individual soldier and the unit, the items of equipment listed below are the primary means of identifying the presence and type of chemicals on the battlefield and determining when a safe condition exists.

- M9 Chemical Agent Detector Paper
- M8 Chemical Agent Detector Paper
- M256A1 Chemical Agent Detector Kit
- Improved Chemical Agent Monitor (ICAM)
- M4A1 Joint Chemical Agent Detector (JCAD)
- M272 Chemical Agent Water Testing Kit
- M22 Automatic Chemical Agent Detector Alarm (ACADA)

M9 Chemical Agent Detector Paper

M9 paper (NSN-6665010498982; TM-3-6665-311-10) is placed on personnel and equipment to detect and identify the presence of liquid nerve or blister agents in exposures as small as 100 μm in diameter. The paper contains an chemical dye that turns pink, red, reddish brown, or red purple when exposed to liquid agents; however, it cannot identify specific agents. M9 paper is manufactured in 30-ft by 2-in adhesive-backed rolls of cream-colored paper. The rolls are packaged with a reusable plastic storage bag in a vacuum-sealed vapor barrier package. The detector paper dye may be a potential carcinogen; chemical protective gloves should be worn when handling M9 paper. Placement of M9 is dictated by the dominant hand of the user. If the user is right-handed, M9 paper should be placed around the right upper arm, left wrist, and right ankle. If the user is left-handed, M9 detector paper should be placed around the left upper arm, right wrist, and left ankle. If a color change is indicated, proper masking, decontamination, and MOPP procedures must be followed.

Although many substances are known to cause false positive responses on M9 paper (antifreeze, liquid insecticide, petroleum products), service members must mask and take other appropriate measures when detection is indicated. Attention to possible interfering substances on the battlefield can help in the later interpretation of a color change on the M9 paper in the absence of confirmation tests for agents.

M8 Chemical Agent Detector Paper

M8 paper (NSN-6665000508529) is used to detect the presence of liquid V-type nerve agents, G-type nerve agents, and H-type blister agents. M8 paper is issued in booklets containing 25 tan-colored sheets of chemically treated dye-impregnated paper. The reverse side of the booklet's front cover contains a color comparison chart for agent recognition. If M8 paper is exposed to chemical agents, the dye-impregnated paper converts from tan to an agent-specific color. Colors corresponding to agents are as follows:

- G-type nonpersistent nerve agents: yellow
- H-type blister agents: red
- V-type persistent nerve agents: olive green or black

If indicated by M8 chemical agent detector paper or encountering a liquid suspected of being a chemical agent, service members must follow proper masking, decontamination, and MOPP procedures. To prepare M8 paper to conduct agent identification, tear one half-sheet from the booklet and affix it to a stick or other object. Using the stick as a handle, blot the paper onto the unknown liquid and wait 30 seconds. Once the 30 seconds has elapsed, compare the sheet to the color comparison chart.

As with M9 paper, M8 paper will show false positive indicators with substances such as antifreeze, liquid insecticide, or petroleum products. Attention to possible interfering substances on the battlefield can help in the later interpretation of a color change on the M8 paper.

M256A1 Chemical Agent Detector Kit

The M256A1 Chemical Agent Detector Kit (NSN-6665011334964; TM-3666530710), designed to detect and identify chemical agents in liquid or vapor, consists of the following:

- A booklet of M8 paper (previously described) to detect agents in liquid form, and
- 12 foil-wrapped detector tickets containing eel enzymes as reagents to detect very low concentrations of chemical vapors.

Table 9-1 lists the agents detected by the M256A1 kit. Instructions for the use of the detector tickets appear on the outside of each of the foil packets and in a separate instruction booklet. By

Table 9-1. Agents Detected by the M256A1 Chemical Agent Detector Kit

Agent	Symbol	Class
Hydrogen cyanide	AC	blood (cyanide)
Cyanogen chloride	CK	blood (cyanide)
Mustard	H	blister
Nitrogen mustard	HN	blister
Distilled mustard	HD	blister
Phosgene oxime	CX	blister
Lewisite	L	blister
Nerve agents	V and G series	nerve

following the directions on the foil packets or in the instruction booklet, service members can conduct a complete test with the liquid-sensitive M8 paper and the vapor-sensitive detector ticket in approximately 20 minutes. During the test, the sampler must be kept out of direct sunlight, which speeds evaporation of the reagents. Waving the detector sampler in the air also accelerates evaporation, so the sampler should be held stationary during all parts of the test.

Improved Chemical Agent Monitor

The ICAM (NSN-6665-01-357-8502; TM-36665343-10) detects agent vapor within a volume of air drawn by the pump into the sampling chamber of the instrument (Figure 9-1). It follows that the inlet port must not come into contact with a suspected area of evaporating agent on a surface but must nevertheless approach within a few inches of the site of suspected contamination. Because of variation in agent concentration from one spot to another, depending upon wind velocity and other environmental factors, numerical displays of agent concentration in typical units would be impractical and unreliable. Accordingly, the display warns of a low vapor hazard (1 to 3 bars visible), a high vapor hazard (4 to 6 bars visible), or a very high vapor hazard (7 to 8 bars visible).

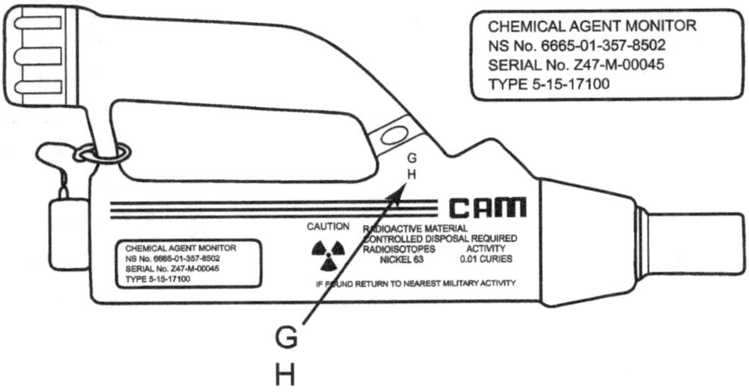

Figure 9-1. Improved Chemical Agent Monitor (ICAM). Used to detect nerve and blister agents as vapors only, the ICAM uses a 10-mCi nickel 63 β-particle radiation source to ionize airborne agent molecules that have been drawn into the unit by a pump. The resulting ion clusters vary in mass and charge and thus also travel at different rates in an applied electrical field. Comparison of the mobility of the different ionic species to electronically stored standards allows an on-board microcomputer to determine the type of agent and its relative concentration. A liquid crystal display presents these data as a series of concentration-dependent bars in a G mode for G agents and VX, and in an H mode for blister agents.

M4A1 Joint Chemical Agent Detector

The JCAD (NSN-6665-01-586-8286; TM 3-6665-456-10) is a hand-held device that automatically detects, identifies, and alerts operators to the presence of nerve and blister vapors, as well as one blood chemical agent vapor and one toxic industrial chemical vapor. The JCAD is modified from a commercially available device and operates as a stand-alone detector. It is capable of supporting the mission requirements of all four services, including:

- interior detection for both tracked and wheeled vehicles,
- fixed- and rotary-wing aircraft interior detection during both ground and airborne operations,
- shipboard interior and exterior detection,

- fixed-site chemical agent detection,
- personal detector to be carried on a individual soldier or used for advanced warning, and
- chemical agent surveys of personnel, equipment, and cargo.

The JCAD can also interface with the Joint Warning and Reporting Network. This interface allows the JCAD to be used as a networked fixed-site detector without direct operator contact. A hasty perimeter network (the Deployable Detector Unit Network function) may be employed through the use of M42 alarm units and WD-1 field wire. Up to ten JCADs may be "strung" together at distances up to 400 m apart. The base unit functions as a control unit to provide chemical alerts and malfunction signals for the other nine deployed units. The JCAD is carried by personnel and placed onto various platforms, including ground vehicles, fixed-site installations, and collective protection shelters.

The detector unit simultaneously detects nerve agents (sarin [GB], tabun [GA], GD, GF, and VX); blister agents (mustard [H], nitrogen mustard [HN3], and lewisite [L]); and blood agents (hydrogen cyanide [AC], cyanogen chloride [CK]). Operating the JCAD in enclosed or poorly ventilated spaces or when sampling near strong vapor sources of the following will sound a false alarm:

- aromatic vapors (eg, aftershave, perfume, food flavorings, peppermint);
- cleaning compounds (eg, disinfectant, menthol, methyl salicylate);
- smoke and fumes and gun oil;
- diesel exhaust, JP-8 (jet fuel) vapor;
- small arms lubricant;
- cigarette smoke; and
- paint fumes and chemical agent-resistant compound.

M22 Automatic Chemical Agent Alarm

The M22 ACADA (NSN-6665-01-438-6963; TM-3-6665-321-12&P) samples the air for the presence of nerve agent (GA, GB, GD) and blister agent (HD, L) vapors, and provides simultaneous detection and warning of these agents (Figure 9-2). It operates

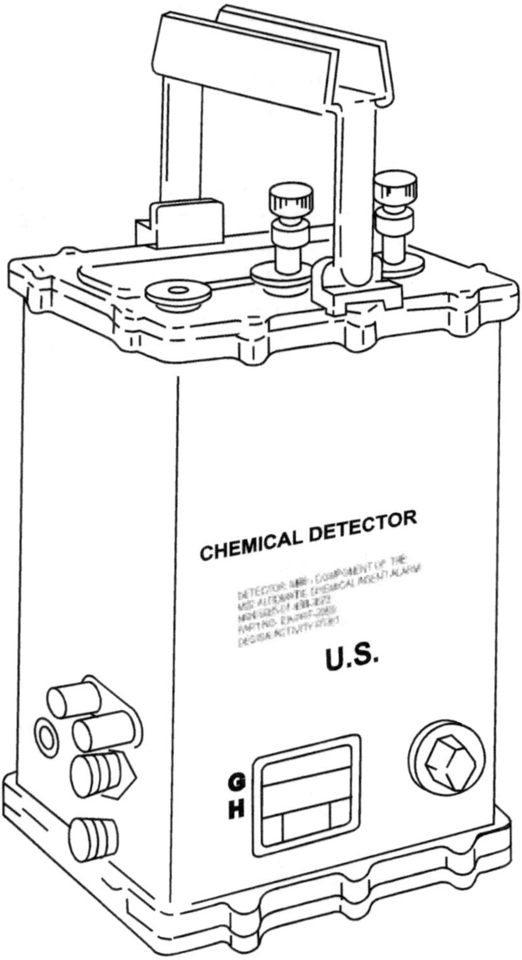

Figure 9-2. The M22 Automatic Chemical Agent Alarm (ACADA), which is capable of detecting and identifying standard blister and nerve agents. The system can be carried by a soldier, operates independently after system start-up, and provides an audible and visual alarm. It also provides communications interface for automatic battlefield warning. The system consists of the M88 detector, as many as five M42 alarm units, a confidence sample, protective caps, square inlet, rain caps, a carrying case, and various power supplies.

in cold and hot climates (- 30°F to 125°F). The following items can interfere with the normal operation of the M22 ACADA and will sound a false alarm:

- tear gas (CS),
- JP-8 jet fuel,
- brake fluid,
- aqueous fire-fighting foam, and
- M18 marking grenades (red and violet).

M272 Chemical Agent Water Testing Kit

The M272 kit (NSN-6665011340885; TM-3666531910) was designed and fielded to answer the need for a test to detect water contamination by nerve agents, blister agents, blood agents (cyanide), and lewisite. The kit will operate between 32°F and 125°F. An enclosed instruction card enables the soldier to conduct all the tests required to identify these threat agents. The kit will detect the chemical agents at the concentrations noted in Table 9-2.

Water containing agents in lesser concentrations than those listed in Table 9-2 is permissible for short-term use (up to 7 days) in both cold and warm regions, as long as the daily consumption per person does not exceed 5 quarts. Each kit contains enough reagents for tests on 25 separate water samples. The operator can easily conduct the full range of tests in 20 minutes when the

Table 9-2. Concentrations of Chemical Agents Detectable by the M272 Chemical Agent Water Testing Kit

Agent	Symbol	Concentration (mg/L)*
Cyanide	AC	20.0 as CN-
Mustard	HD	2.0
Lewisite	L	2.0 as As+++
Nerve agents	G, V	0.02

*Concentration reliably detected by kit tests. CN- is the liquid form of cyanide measurable in water.
As+++ is a form of arsenic, the positive elemental ion arsenous, which is measurable in water.

temperature is between 50°F and 105°F; at lower temperatures, the water samples and the nerve agent ticket should both be warmed for 10 minutes before beginning testing. Water that is too hot may cause foaming in the detector tubes for lewisite, mustard, and cyanide; therefore, water at temperatures between 105°F and 125°F should be cooled for at least 5 minutes to reduce its temperature to 105°F or cooler.

Patient Protective Equipment

This section discusses the following items:
- Patient Protective Wrap Kit
- Decontaminable Litter
- Resuscitation Device, Individual Chemical (RDIC)

Patient Protective Wrap Kit

Decontamination and medical treatment of chemical casualties often requires clothing removal and precludes dressing them in replacement JSLIST. The Patient Protective Wrap (PPW) Kit (NSN-6545-01-577-1047) was developed as an alternative form of protection. When used in conjunction with the consumable items listed below, the wrap protects uncontaminated patients from potential contamination during evacuation. The PPW protects the patient from exposure to harmful chemical and biological materials for up to 6 continuous hours. It consists of two components: the protective wrap and a motor blower assembly. Resembling a lightweight sleeping bag, the wrap is 107 cm wide by 249 cm long and weighs 2.7 kg. It is fabricated of a carbon-impregnated permeable top sheet and impermeable bottom sheet that is unaffected by all bodily fluids. The top sheet has an impermeable transparent window to permit observation of the patient. A protected entryway for inserting intravenous tubing is located at each side of the window. The blower is a small, lightweight unit providing a continuous flow of clean, filtered breathing air, which considerably reduces the danger of heat stress on the casualty, and increases the operational effectiveness of the wrap in hot climates.

NOTE: Patients should not be left in the wrap longer than 6 hours.

Decontaminable Litter

Contaminated casualties arriving at a medical treatment location will in most cases require decontamination prior to definitive treatment. The decontamination process requires the use of equipment organic to the treatment unit. Ideally, any equipment in limited supply should be capable of complete decontamination using field-available methods. The Decontaminable Litter (NSN 6530-01-290-9964) is made from a monofilament polypropylene that has high tensile strength and low elasticity. The fabric does not absorb liquid chemical agents and is not degraded by decontaminating solutions. It is flame retardant, highly rip resistant, and treated to withstand exposure to weather and sunlight. The fabric has a honeycomb weave, which results in a rough, non-slip surface, and liquids easily pass through the 40% of surface area that is open. The litter has carrying handles that retract into the metal pole frame for a closed total length of 83.5 in (212.1 cm) to allow the litter to be loaded onto the UH-60 helicopter. The handles have two open carrying positions: 90.0 in (228.1 cm) and 91.6 in (232.7 cm). The first position is a NATO standard; the second position allows increased gripping comfort. The aluminum poles were designed to provide direct gripping surfaces for litter stanchions. All metal parts are painted with chemical agent-resistant coating paint.
NOTE: Canvas litters exposed to liquid blister agents and then decontaminated still desorbed vapors for 72 hours.

Resuscitation Device, Individual Chemical

The Resuscitation Device, Individual Chemical (RDIC; NSN 6515-01-338-6602) is a ventilatory system consisting of a compressible butyl rubber bag, a NATO standard C2 canister filter, a non-rebreathing valve, a cricothyroid cannula adapter, and a flexible hose connected to an oropharyngeal mask. The mask is removable from the distal end of the flexible hose to allow the hose to be connected to the cannula adapter. The butyl rubber bag resists the penetration of liquid chemical agent that may be on the operator's chemical protective gloves, and is easily decontaminated. The elasticity of the outer cover limits airway pressure to a maximal value of 70 cm H_2O. The device will deliver up to 600 mL of filtered air per cycle at a rate of 30 cycles per minute. The RDIC is used in a contaminated environment to ventilate casualties.

Appendix A

PATIENT DECONTAMINATION STATION DIAGRAMS

The following diagrams show set-up for casualty management in a contaminated environment. Chapter 8, on casualty management, describes the various areas. The actual set-up of this station may vary depending on circumstances and available assets.

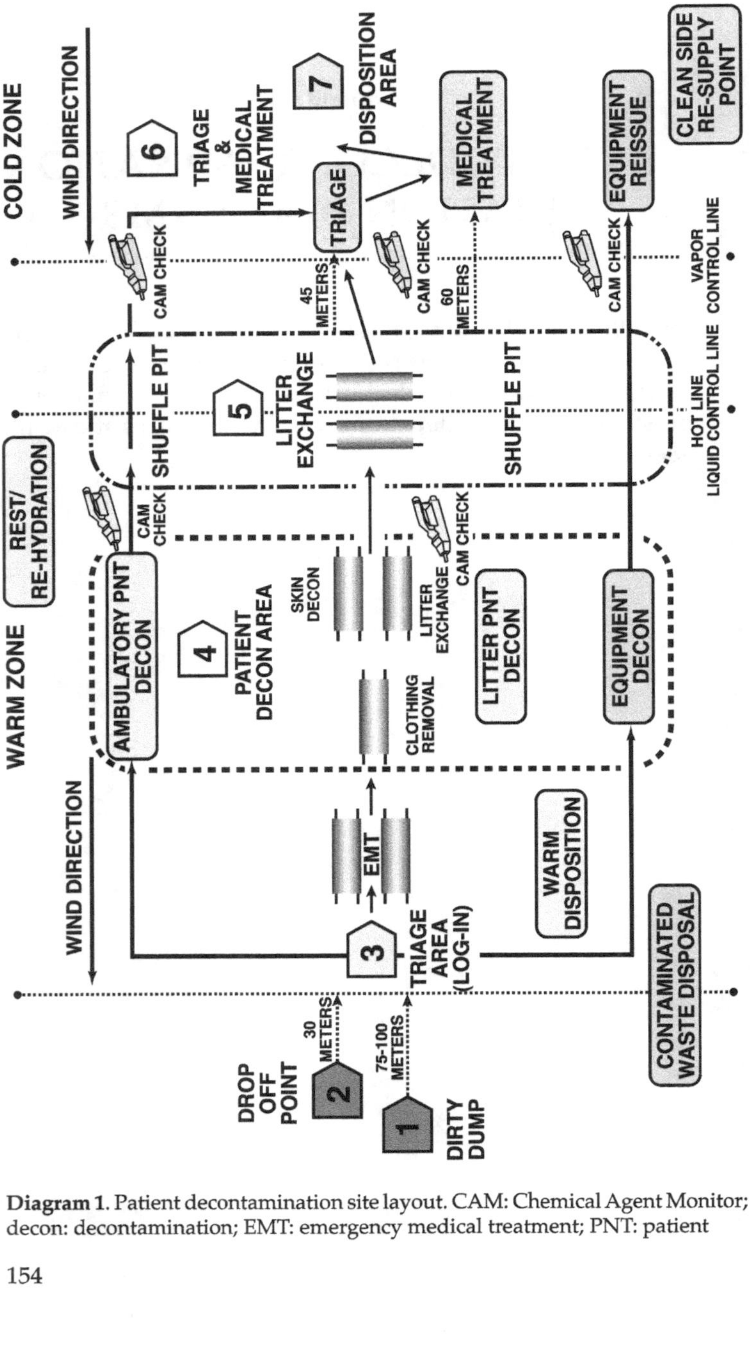

Diagram 1. Patient decontamination site layout. CAM: Chemical Agent Monitor; decon: decontamination; EMT: emergency medical treatment; PNT: patient

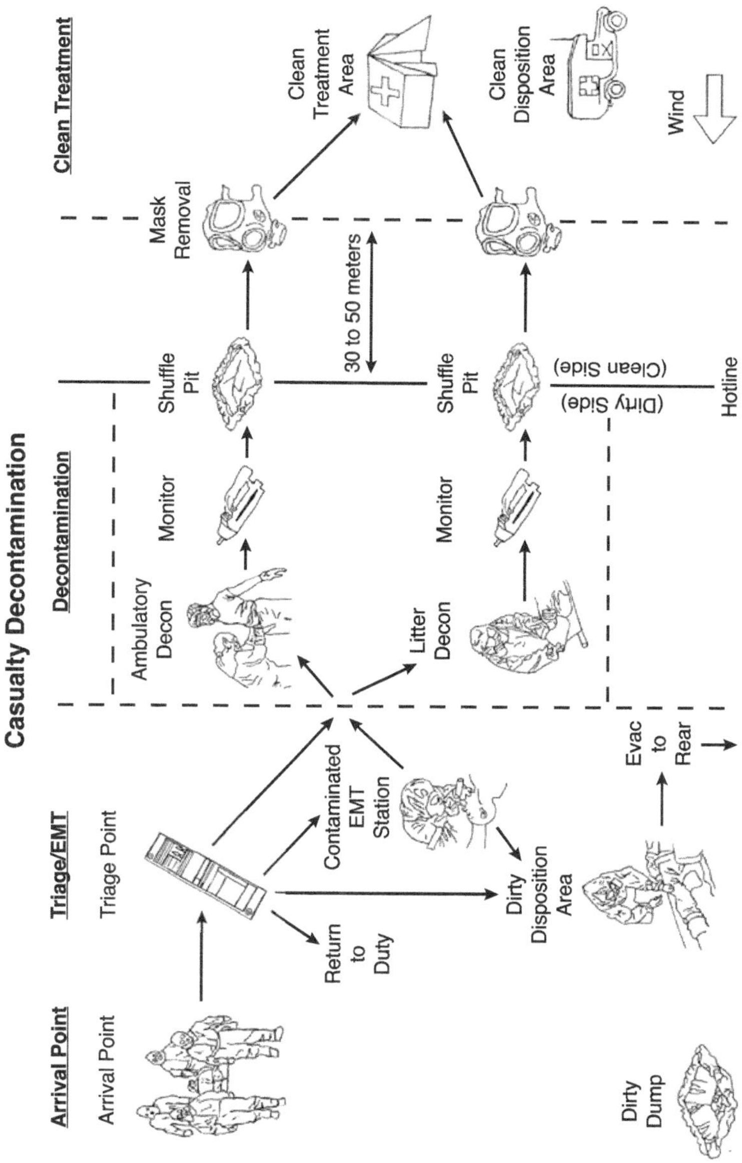

Diagram 2. Casualty decontamination procedure. EMT: emergency medical treatment

Appendix B

PHYSIOCHEMICAL DATA

The following table provides physiochemical data on the agents discussed in this handbook.

Agent	Molecular Weight	Vapor Density (Compared to Air)	Liquid Density (g/mL)
GA *Tabun*	162	5.63	1.07 @ 25°C
GB *Sarin*	140	4.86	1.102 @ 20°C
GF	180	6.2	1.17 @ 20°C
GD *Soman*	182	6.33	1.02 @ 25°C
VX	267	9.2	1.01 @ 20°C
HD *Distilled mustard*	159	5.4	1.27 @ 20°C
L *Lewisite*	207	7.1	1.89 @ 20°C
CX *Phosgene oxime*	114	3.9	NA
AC *Hydrogen cyanide*	27	0.94	0.94
CK *Cyanogen choride*	61.5	2.1	1.18
CG *Phosgene*	99	3.4	1.37
CN *Mace*	154.59	5.3	1.32 (solid) @ 20°C
CS	189	NA	1.04 @ 20°C

*HD decomposes before boiling at 218°C. HD as a liquid will still boil, but the agent decomposes (HD is demilitarized in a similar process).
NA: not available

Freezing/ Melting Point (°C)	Boiling Point (°C @ 750 mm HG)	Vapor Pressure (mm HG @ 25°C)	Volatility (mg/m³ @ 25°C)
- 50	247	0.07	610
- 56	147	2.9	17,000
- 30	239 (@ 20°C)	0.04 (@ 20°C)	581
- 42	167	0.4	3,900
- 39	298	0.0007	10
14.5	227.8*	0.07 @ 20°C	600 @ 20°C
-1 8	190	0.2239 @ 20°C	4,480 @ 20°C
35–40	128	11.2 @ 25°C	1,800 @ 20°C
- 13.3	25.7	630 @ 20°C	1,080,000 @ 25°C
- 6.9	12.8	1,230 @2 5°C	2,600,000 @ 12.8°C
-1 28	7.6	1.17 @ 20°C	4,300,000 @ 7.6°C
58	248	0.0041 @ 20°C	115 @ 20°C
- 94	315	0.00034 @ 20°C	0.71 @ 20°C

Appendix C

CHEMICAL AGENT QUICK REFERENCE

The following table is intended to serve as a quick reference of chemical agents, their effects, first-aid measures, detection, and skin decontamination. Consult the appropriate chapter for further details.

Type of Agent	Effects	Onset
Pulmonary TICs: CG, PFIB, HC	Dyspnea, coughing	Hours
Cyanide: AC, CK	Loss of consciousness, convulsions, apnea	Seconds
Vesicants: H, HD, L	Liquid: erythema, blisters; irritation of eyes; cough, dyspnea. Vapor: miosis, rhinorrhea, dyspnea	Liquid: hours (immediate pain after L). Vapor: seconds
Nerve agents: GA, GB, GD, GF, VX	Liquid: sweating, vomiting. Vapor: miosis, rhinorrhea, dyspnea. Both: convulsions, apnea	Liquid: minutes to hours. Vapor: seconds
Incapacitating agents: BZ, Agent 15	Mydriasis, increased body temperature; dry mouth and skin; confusion; visual hallucinations	Minutes to hours
Riot-control agents: CS, CN	Burning, stinging of eyes, nose, airways, skin	Seconds

ACADA: Automatic Chemical Agent Detection Alarm
ATNAA: Antidote Treatment Nerve Agent Autoinjector
ICAM: Improved Chemical Agent Monitor
JCAD: Joint Chemical Agent Detector
PFIB: perfluoroisobutylene
RSDL: Reactive Skin Decontamination Lotion
TIC: toxic industrial chemical

First-aid	Skin Decontamination	Field Detection
None	None usually needed	None
None (nitrite and thiosulfate)	None usually needed	JCAD, M256A1, M18A2
None	RSDL, soap and water, 0.5% hypochlorite solution	JCAD, M256A1; M8 and M9 papers, ICAM, ACADA, FOX, M90
ATNAA (1 to 3); diazepam	RSDL, soap and water, 0.5% hypochlorite solution	JCAD, M256A1, M8 and M9 papers, ICAM, M22 ACADA
Prevent casualties from harming themselves or others	Remove outer clothing; water or soap and water	None
None	Water	None

Appendix D

NEMONICS

The ABCDDs of Chemical Casualty Care

A: Airway management should be focused on establishing an airway and maintaining the airway. Death will occur if the airway is lost.

B: Breathing may require intubation and ventilation of casualties. Keep in mind that once a casualty has been intubated, someone must stay with the casualty to provide and monitor ventilations. This requirement may last until evacuation or return of spontaneous breathing, or until the patient expires.

C: Circulation: to maintain circulation in the absence of effective cardiac contractions, chest compressions may be required but will probably not be feasible in a mass-casualty event. Most casualties without a pulse will have to be triaged as expectant.

D: Decontamination: immediate, along with thorough patient decontamination and technical decontamination, constitutes one of the main types of personnel decontamination.

D: Drugs: refers to specific antidotal treatment for selected agents and also to ancillary supportive medications.

Toxicology Acronyms

Acronyms are helpful for remembering the toxicologically important aspects of a poisoned casualty. Choose the one that you find easiest to remember and commit it to memory. The logical progression of each acronym from agent through environment and to host should aid memorization.

ASBESTOS

A: Agent(s): type(s) and estimated doses
S: State(s): solid, liquid, vapor, gas, aerosol
B: Body sites: where exposed (routes of entry, exposure and absorption)
E: Effects: local vs systemic
S: Severity: of effects and exposure
T: Time course: past, present, and future (prognosis)
O: Other diagnoses: instead of (differential diagnosis) and in addition to (additional diagnoses)
S: Synergism: interaction among multiple coexisting diagnoses

TOXICANT

T: Toxicant/toxidrome: does the agent fit with a specific toxidrome?
O: Outside the body: is its form solid, liquid, vapor, gas, or aerosol?
X: Xing into the body: where did the agent cross into the body (exposure and absorption)?
I: Inside the body: where did the agent go inside the body (distribution)?
C: Chronology: what is the time course of exposure (past, present, and future)?
A: Additional diagnoses: are there coexisting diagnoses?
N: Net effect of diagnoses: what is the effect of the interaction among all diagnoses, on the patient as a whole?
T: Triage: what is the patient's priority for treatment, decontamination, and transport?

POISON

P: Poison(s): what are the type(s) and estimated doses?
O: Outside the body: is the agent solid, liquid, vapor, gas, or aerosol?
I: Into/inside the body: where did it get into the body and where did it go inside the body?
S: Sequence of events: what is the time course off effects (past, present, and future)?
O: Other diagnoses: are there other causes, instead of (differential diagnosis) and in addition to (additional diagnoses)?
N: Net effects of diagnoses: what results from the interaction among all diagnoses, for the patient as a whole?

Appendix E

GLOSSARY OF TERMS AND ACRONYMS

ABCs. airway, breathing, circulation
ABCDDs. Airway, Breathing, Circulation, immediate Decontamination, and Drugs
ACAA. Automatic Chemical Agent Alarm
ACADA. Automatic Chemical Agent Detector Alarm; this area monitoring detector sounds a warning when it senses the vapors of blister and nerve agents
Acid. a substance with a pH less than 7
ACU. Army combat uniform
AFS. Alternative Footwear Solution
Aerosol. a gaseous suspension of fine solid or liquid particles
Alkali. a substance with a pH greater than 7
Alveoli. microscopic air sacs in the lungs where oxygen and carbon dioxide diffusion (movement) takes place through alveolar walls
AMEDD. Army Medical Department
Asphyxiation. unconsciousness or death caused by lack of oxygen
ATNAA. Antidote Treatment Nerve Agent Autoinjector
BAL. British anti-Lewisite
Bronchi. the finer, smaller divisions of the wind pipe as it enters the lungs
BSA. body surface area
C2A1 filter canister. the standard filter used on the military mask; protects against historical chemical warfare agents
CAM. Chemical Agent Monitor
CANA. Convulsive Antidote, Nerve Agent.
Capillaries. small blood vessels
CARC. Chemical Agent-Resistant Coating
Central airway. the airway segment that transports air from the nose and mouth to the lungs

CNS. central nervous system
Ct. concentration-time product
CWC. Chemical Warfare Convention
ECP. entry control point
ED_{50}. effective dose
EEG. electroencephalographic
EMT. emergency medical treatment
FiO_2. fraction of inspired oxygen
FMC. Field Medical Card
FR. flame-resistant
nFR. non–flame-resistant
GCSF. granulocyte colony stimulating factor
GI. gastrointestinal
HC smoke. military tactical smoke
HEPA. high-efficiency particulate air
HTH. high test hypochlorite
ICAD. Individual Chemical Agent Detector
ICAM. Improved Chemical Agent Monitor
Intubation. the process of enhancing respiration by providing an artificial airway
ICt_{50}. median incapacitating dose via vapor
ID_{50}. median incapacitating dose
IDLH. immediately dangerous to life and health
IM. intramuscular
IP. intraperitoneal
IPE. individual protective equipment
IV. intravenous
JB2GU. Joint Block 2 Glove Upgrade
JCAD. Joint Chemical Agent Detector
JSGPM. Joint Service General Purpose Mask
JSLIST. Joint Service Lightweight Integrated Suit Technology
JSPDS. Joint Service Personnel/Skin Decontamination System
L. lewisite
Laryngospasm. spasmodic closure of the larynx (voice box at the top of the trachea/wind pipe)
Larynx. voicebox and vocal cords
LCL. liquid control line
LCt_{50}. median lethal concentration
LD_{50}. median lethal dose

LSD. lysergic acid diethylamide
MCBC. Management of Chemical and Biological Casualties course
MCW. mass-casualty weapon
MES. medical equipment set
MOPP. mission-oriented protective posture
MTF. medical treatment facility
Nasopharynx. the area of the nose and upper airway
NATO. North Atlantic Treaty Organization
NBC. nuclear/biological/chemical
NCO. noncommissioned officer
NCOIC. noncommissioned officer-in-charge
NOx. oxides of nitrogen; toxic smoke that can cause pulmonary edema. Produced by exploding munitions, industrial smoke, and in grain silos as a product of grain fermentation
OIC. officer-in-charge
Oropharynx. the mouth and upper airway
OSHA. Occupational Safety and Health Agency
PDS. patient decontamination site
PFIB. toxic smoke produced by Teflon (DuPont, Wilmington, DE) burning at over 700°F
PNS. peripheral nervous system
PO. per os (by mouth)
PPW. Patient Protective Wrap
Pulmonary edema. fluid in the lungs, associated with an outpouring of fluids from the capillaries into the pulmonary spaces (air sacs or alveoli) producing severe shortness of breath. In later stages, produces expectoration of frothy, pink, fluid and blue lips (cyanosis)
RDD. radiological dispersal device
RDIC. Resuscitation Device, Individual Chemical
RSCAAL. Remote Sensing Chemical Agent Alarm
RSDL. Reactive Skin Decontamination Lotion
TAP. toxicological agent protective (eg, TAP apron)
TIB. toxic industrial biological
TIC. toxic industrial chemical; a chemical with a toxicity equal to or greater than ammonia that is produced more than 30 times a year by an industrial facility
TIM. toxic industrial material

TIR. toxic industrial radiological
Trachea. wind pipe
USAMRICD. US Army Medical Research Institute of Chemical Defense
Vapor. fumes given off by a liquid
VCL. vapor control line
WBGT. wet bulb globe thermometer
WMDs. weapons of mass destruction

INDEX

D

J

L

M

U

V

W

Z

www.ingramcontent.com/pod-product-compliance
Lightning Source LLC
Chambersburg PA
CBHW070742180526
45167CB00012B/1871